Celia Wright writes regularly for *Living* magazine and contributes to several other women's magazines. She and Brian Wright started the Green Farm Nutrition Centre in 1979, in Sussex, to pioneer the 'new nutrition' in Britain. The idea that nutrition itself could be used for healing was little understood when they began, and the information needed for this natural healing process was not publicly available. By offering a nationwide membership and magazine, running information and consultation services by post, offering courses, cassette tapes and books, but above all, by seeding their ideas into numerous magazine articles and local radio and television programmes, the Wrights have succeeded in helping to bring nutritional consciousness to the public eye.

CELIA WRIGHT

The Wright Diet

GRAFTON BOOKS

A Division of the Collins Publishing Group

LONDON GLASGOW
TORONTO SYDNEY AUCKLAND

Grafton Books
A Division of the Collins Publishing Group
8 Grafton Street, London W1X 3LA

Published by Grafton Books 1989

First published in Great Britain by
Judy Piatkus (Publishers) Ltd 1986

ISBN 0-586-20408-3

Printed and bound in Great Britain by
Collins, Glasgow

Set in Times

Acknowledgements

I should like to express my gratitude and appreciation to the following people for their advice, help and support during the writing of this book: Brian Wright, David Simpson, Monica Bryant, Penny Davenport, Carole Simpson, Timothy Wilson, Caroline Shaw, Rosemary and Robert Paice, Kate Weaver, Helena Weaver, all the staff of the Green Farm Nutrition Centre, Christina Dodwell, Ben Page, Dr Richard Beale, Dr R. Schoental, Jeffrey Bland Ph.D., Dr H. Sinclair, Professor Michael Crawford, Dr Richard Turner, to my agent Maggie Noach, to Judy Piatkus, Hetty Thistlethwaite, and Gill Cormode of Piatkus Books (for their patience!), to Dena Vane and Jackie Highe of *Living* magazine, and to Mozart, Steve Winwood, Jean Michel Jarre and Phil Collins for keeping me company through the nights.

Contents

PART THREE
The Right Food

PART ONE
The Wright Diet

1

The Healthiest Diet In The World

I am probably the most unlikely person to be writing about health and nutrition. I don't come from a background of grapefruit, brisk walks and nut rissoles at all. In fact I grew up on an appalling diet of chips, white bread and chocolates. Worse than that I have a self-indulgent nature. I don't say no to myself; I never could.

On the other hand you could say that all this makes me the perfect person for the job. For ten years I've been working on a diet for optimum health that also allows you to feel good while you're doing it. Understanding human temptation only too well (I was trained as a psychologist) I've developed a diet that works with human nature and not against it.

Nevertheless the way that you feel about food is going to change radically. On the Wright Diet you're going to lose all those old cravings, and quite naturally develop a taste for nutritious, satisfying and health-enhancing foods. When you're on the Wright Diet you won't need to say no to yourself either.

The Wright Diet is the healthiest diet in the world. Not only that. It's the only diet you can change to suit you perfectly. There is *no one right diet* that suits everyone. Each of us is slightly different; we each have different nutritional needs. There is no diet, however healthy, that can be right for all of us. Except the Wright Diet.

This is how it works. First, the Wright Diet gives you high level health in these ten ways:

1 High Fibre
The Wright Diet is high in the unprocessed foods on which our ancestors thrived for millennia.

2 Low to Very Low Fat
Depending on your food choices, the Wright Diet is either low or very low in fat. The fats and oils that you do eat on the diet actually protect your heart and circulation, and benefit your skin and health too.

3 Sugar-Free
Delicious sugar-free recipes to keep down your weight, *and* keep your sweet tooth happy.

4 Salt-Free
Food full of flavour yet with no excess sodium. The Wright Diet protects your heart and your blood pressure, and helps prevent water retention.

5 Acid/Alkaline Balance
A high alkaline diet for health and self-healing, for inner calm and for steady emotions.

6 Blood Sugar Balance
The Wright Diet gives you steady and balanced blood sugar for freedom from depression and from cravings, and for maximum strength and energy.

7 50 Per Cent Raw Foods
A high raw food diet packed with vitamins, minerals, enzymes and alkalinity.

8   Free of Cooking Dangers
On the Wright Diet you cook simply and avoid the ageing and cancer-provoking effects of some forms of cookery.

9   The Right Food Combinations
The Wright Diet guides you to the food combinations that work best for digestion, and your personal health needs.

10   The Right Food Supplements
An optional Basic Supplement Programme to safeguard your immunity and promote high level health.

These ten health factors alone give you a higher possibility of health than any other diet yet written, but the Wright Diet doesn't stop there.

It gives you the widest possible selection of healthy foods to choose from, as well as the method you need to find exactly which foods are healthy for you. With the Wright Diet you can build your own right diet.

This has enormous repercussions for your well-being. For the first time there is a diet, based on the most up to date information, that can help you work out which foods will heal your body. Eating grains and not cheese, for instance, could put an end to your headaches. Eating oats but not bread could save you from years of depression. Giving up eggs, or eating more fish might heal a chronic skin condition. Cutting down on all dairy products might end your premenstrual tension.

The results will be different for each of us; none of these tactics would work for everyone. But the Wright Diet will tell you exactly which changes in diet are right for your body. When you know that, you will find a level of health you have never experienced before.

There is no other diet that can do this. All other diets

tie up your options. Vegetarian foods are healthy for some, but not if your body can't handle nuts, cheese and lentils. The high protein diets work for others, but not if meat is too heavy for your digestion. The F Plan may fill you up with lots of healthy fibre, but some of us don't tolerate wheat bran. Macrobiotic foods can also be health-giving, but not if you have a problem with salt, grains and pulses. And the allergy diets may help you to discover the foods you can't handle, but don't prescribe other foods that are necessarily healthy at all.

Only the Wright Diet can give you all the health principles rolled into one enjoyable process. Once you've started, you'll wonder why you ever ate differently.

Seduced by Health

My path from sugar to salads began quite unexpectedly one summer in the seventies. In the hot London summer of 1976 I got involved in a project with fellow professionals running a café in the King's Road.

We served a lot of healthy salads at the café, but we also did a roaring trade in cheesecake. Since none of us had ever run a café before (the project was really more about teamwork than food) we were all pretty stretched. We made up for it by grabbing quick slabs of cheesecake, endless cups of strong black coffee, and Marlborough cigarettes from the machine on the wall.

One night at a cinema with Brian Wright, a fellow psychologist, I became aware of an acute pain under my right ribcage, so intense that it took my breath away. From what I know now I would say that I was passing a gallstone, brought on by the very high fat content of my cheesecake diet. The pain eventually passed, but the sense that all was not well did not.

Shortly afterwards Brian and I moved away from the

café and went to live close to Wimbledon Common. We spent a great deal of our time together walking on the Common and sharing our ideas. Slowly a growing consciousness of our need for health emerged from all this. Perhaps it was all that green and fresh air after living for so long in the city.

Instinctively we gave up smoking and began to eat more salads. We even cut down on our sugar intake, generally getting more wholefood-conscious. And there I think we might have stayed, as do most people who get a little concerned about their health. But fate had something much more drastic in store for us. The American nutritionist Marshall Lever was in London for a few weeks and friends suggested, since we were interested, that we should consult him. He gave us both individual nutritional programmes to follow that included nutritional supplements and a radical change of diet.

I could not have been more astonished with the result. Quantitatively it was the biggest change in my well-being that I had yet experienced. From feeling exhausted, achy, and more than a little disillusioned after so many years of searching for answers, I found myself running and leaping with delight because I felt so good. All the hard work that I had put in up till that point showed too, of course, but I knew that I had just found a missing link.

Nutritional Discoveries
Nutritional healing, at that time in this country, was almost unheard of. The kind of service Marshall Lever had offered us in his brief stay in London was practically unique. The official line of the medical profession and government departments was that vitamins were needed in trace amounts to correct deficiency diseases, and these were practically non-existent in our now well-fed society.

About the use of food for healing there were no guidelines at all – the idea that food itself could be used for healing wasn't even considered as a possibility. The practice of 'naturopathy' did exist among some alternative practitioners but it was thirty years out of date and contained none of the innovative ideas that had done so much for us.

We set to work to understand just how the diets we had been given had worked. We searched through medical physiology and the medical and scientific literature for the connections we were looking for. The scraps of evidence were few and far between at first. For much of the time we only had the evidence of our own experience to keep us going. But as the months passed we started to piece together a picture. Files full of papers from the medical journals grew alongside the feedback we were getting from the people who were now coming to us for help with their own nutrition.

Within three years we had received hundreds of letters and phone calls and had moved to an old farmhouse near Burwash in Sussex, called Green Farm. We started a small business in the nutrition area that would keep us funded while we continued our work, and opened Green Farm membership to those seriously interested in nutritional healing. It was soon a thousand strong and the letters kept pouring in. They have never stopped.

Now we have a centre called the Green Farm Nutrition Centre where we have the space to give courses and consultations, and room for the staff and offices that our enterprise now requires. In an average year we receive over twelve thousand letters and calls. We also get constant attention from the media – requests for us to write articles and diets, for interviews, for television and radio slots, and for contributions to books. We get the feeling that nutritional healing is coming into its own.

A Diet for Health
In 1980 I met Leslie Kenton of *Harpers and Queen*. We had exchanged letters because each of us was interested in what the other was doing. I really admired the pioneering nutritional journalism that Leslie had been doing (she was also interested in raw foods and was planning her recent book at the time), and Leslie was very interested in some of our ideas and approaches to nutritional healing. When we met at the *Harpers and Queen* offices, Leslie asked if I would like to try my hand at writing a diet for the magazine using the Green Farm principles of nutrition.

Although I'd written a small paperback called the Nutrition Handbook which we'd published privately, I had never considered writing anything for the public at large. 'Diet' to me meant serious nutrition, but now I was being asked to produce something in the format of a magazine diet. But this time with a difference – this time it would be a diet that would really do something for the people who tried it. 'Make it a rejuvenating diet,' Leslie said, 'something that will really help cleanse and regenerate the body.' With difficulty I condensed my ideas on diet into a workable nine-day format. We called it 'The Nine Days to a New Woman Diet.'

The diet was an extraordinary success. People from all over the world wrote to say that the diet had made them feel marvellous, or cured their cystitis, or helped them lose weight, or helped them sleep, or a hundred different things. I was amazed and thrilled. It had been a marvellous opportunity to get wider feedback on the ideas I was using, and the feedback had been good. Soon I was being asked to write diets for other national magazines. Then I wrote a carefully thought-out weight loss diet for the magazine we now call the *Green Farm Magazine*. There was also a version for healing skin and hair conditions.

The Wright Diet
I called this one the Wright Diet. I doubt if that issue went to more than two thousand people, but one of them happened to be the journalist Anne Hooper. Unknown to me she put her family on to the Wright Diet straight away. One day she phoned to say would it be okay to put a small mention in *Cosmopolitan* that readers could obtain a reprint of the diet if they sent us 30p? Of course we said yes, and promptly forgot about it.

Four or five months later we were taking a rare holiday when a friend came out to join us. Back home, she told us, the Nutrition Centre was practically under siege. A whole glowing article on my diet had appeared in *Cosmopolitan* and requests for offprints together with 30p in coins, stamps and goodness knows what else, were coming in by the sackload!

When we got home we saw what she meant. It was taking the entire staff of the Nutrition Centre, then some six people, the whole morning of every day to open the mail. Overall we had about six or seven thousand requests. In the end we lost count, and even now, some three years later, we still get requests from *Cosmopolitan* readers.

In the months that followed, the feedback letters started to come in. One woman wrote:

'Now more than one year has passed since I started your Wright Diet plan. I lost the kilos I wanted to and I'm still this way. The gastritis I suffered has subsided.

I used to suffer depression but now I feel fine. I've never been depressed again even in difficult situations.'

And another:

'I have had psoriasis of the scalp for the past 6½ years and am now 18½ years old, the condition having continually worsened. I must admit I held out no hope of the regime working but decided it was worth a try. May I say how pleased I am now that I did. There is a most rewarding improvement. Several patches have disappeared completely, normal scalp is showing in small places on the main area and this is also shrinking in size. The build up is very much reduced too.'

And one which gave me particular pleasure, as tough cases always do:

'I was delighted to read your article about people who find it very difficult, almost impossible to lose weight on conventional diets. I was beginning to think I was a "freak". Reading through your article I realised I fitted into all three categories listed and as diet instructions devised by yourself were given I decided to embark on this new diet.
'Through my 20 years of dieting I have gone through most diets without lasting success and have developed a deep-rooted obsession about overweight. I have even gone so far as to consult a hypnotherapist who after 6 sessions declared I cannot be helped by hypnotherapy. I am regularly treated/checked by a natural therapist who can't pinpoint the cause of the trouble either.
'On the 4th of January I started your diet weighing 13

*stone and have, to date (18th February), lost 1 stone 5
lbs which I think is absolutely miraculous.'*

After this success friends started to urge me to write up
the Wright Diet as a book. But I didn't do it then, and
I'm glad that I didn't because my ideas have changed a lot
since then. The book I would have written then would not
have contained many ideas I now know to be essential.
Like other writers I started out with fixed ideas about
which diets were right and which were wrong. Over the
years my clients and my own body have taught me to
think otherwise. There can only be one right diet and that
is the one that helps you to find the best diet for yourself.
That is the Wright Diet.

Using this book
In Chapters 2 and 3, I give you the background to the diet
and how it works. There isn't any mystery about this.
Everything has full scientific backing. If you're interested
you'll find all the references to the scientific papers and
literature that support the diet at the back of the book.

Then Chapter 4 tells you what you need to know about
your body. The Wright Diet will be of most use to you
when you can tell what's actually happening to your body
when you eat.

After that you're ready for the diet itself in Chapter 5.
There's a special seven-day diet to get you going, followed
by a regular routine. On the Wright Diet you have days
when you can feast (and eat whatever you like), as well
as days of fruit fasting and simple healthy eating. The diet
as a whole will bring about healing, weight loss and
cleansing while remaining a regime that you can happily
stick to for ever.

Chapter 6 explains the Food Tests, a simple way of

varying the Wright Diet to find out exactly which foods work well for you and which don't.

In Part Two I explain how you can use the Wright Diet for healing; for increasing energy or getting a good night's sleep; for getting over cravings and losing weight; for dealing with women's problems; for improving your skin and holding on to your hair; for getting over depression; getting rid of headaches, and so on.

Part Three gives you the recipes and a whole set of food charts and advice for the kitchen. By then you should have everything you need to find your own right diet.

IMPORTANT NOTE This book cannot and does not attempt to diagnose your health problems or prescribe for them. If you are concerned about your health you should see a doctor.

2
The Lost Instinct

I sometimes feel that my ideas about food are so straight-forward – such obvious extensions of common sense – that I hardly need explain them. Then I take a look at the food diaries that my clients bring me, or I make a rare dash into a supermarket for bin liners or shoelaces, and I glimpse with horror at what is going into everyone else's baskets. There can only be one explanation for the suicidal feeding habits I see around me. *People have totally lost their instincts as to how to feed themselves.*

I'm frequently approached by people who want to know if I think they should eat meat (or citrus fruit, or yoghurt, or whatever). Or they write in distress that several nutritional authors have completely opposing views, so would I add my view to help them make up their mind? Or they tell me that they eat nothing but tea and biscuits and can I suggest how they can improve their diet?

I have views on all these questions of course, but I cannot tell anyone what or how to eat – I can only make suggestions. On the contrary it is they who should be able to tell me – their body alone knows what it needs. Questions like these again indicate that people have lost touch with a vital and natural instinct, and are left with very little idea of what they really need.

No one reading this book should ever need to ask such questions again. Not because I give the answers. But because what the Wright Diet will do for you is reconnect you with that instinct about your body and how to feed it, so that you will 'know' the answers to such questions for yourself. That doesn't mean of course that you don't need to learn the principles in the first place. You do. But what you need even more is the ability to be able to digest and assess whatever is being said and then check it out for yourself. Because taking anyone's word (including my own) as gospel, is no way to know anything.

Where did that lost instinct go? What is it that reduces people to confused and poorly nourished impulse-feeders who stuff their mouths with biscuits, instant suppers and chemical pickle? And what can we do to get that instinct back once we realise that we've lost it?

Our Tastes are Fooled

One clue to what has happened may be illustrated by quoting the approach used in TV advertisements. 'The family will go crazy for this!' they say. But how many people realise that this claim may literally be *true*? Modern processed foods are very big business. They are deliberately peppered with addictive chemicals (some food additives are now known to be addictive[1]) – precisely because people will go mad for them and their sales will rocket.

After all the food manufacturers are not primarily in business to produce food. They exist to make profits. So any ingredient that boosts sales will automatically be stepped up. And real foods don't produce cravings and empty the shelves. Can you imagine the family screaming for more and more natural yoghurt? Or plain boiled potato? No, it's the artificial 'fruit' flavoured yoghurt, the synthetic desserts and the phoney crisps that can make grovelling idiots of us all.

Small wonder I get letters that say, 'Please help me, I am absolutely desperate. I don't know any more how to eat, what to eat, or when to eat.'

But it isn't just additives that have eroded our natural

instincts. One of my early addictions was to salted crisps. Crisps are salted of course because who'd go mad for cold sliced potato without it? Salt has been used for centuries as a preservative. Now it's redundant. We have fridges and freezers instead. But many people still take in twenty times their daily requirement of sodium (salt)[2] *because they're actually addicted to it.*

Salt, and of course sugar, are two of the oldest taste-distorters known to man. Either one will deceive our tastebuds so much that we will eat (and even crave) total rubbish – including in some cases total non-foods such as toothpaste – so long as the taste is sweet or salty enough.

Most of us have more sense about refuelling our cars than we do our bodies. We habitually let ourselves run out of energy by eating the wrong foods at the wrong meals (high sugar breakfasts for instance, or inadequate lunches), or by going too long without eating at all. Then we're forced to refuel quickly under emergency conditions. That's when we load up with chocolate, sweets, sticky buns, and sugary cups of coffee and tea – none of which are really food at all.

But all these short-term fuel-boosters do is make you hungry again. They're so sweet they force the body to make extra insulin, the hormone that takes fuel out of the bloodstream and stores it in the muscles. Once again our instincts are totally fooled. Very soon we're hungry again and we feel driven to reach for another bar of chocolate or a biscuit (to quickly refuel the bloodstream), instead of getting something nourishing to eat.

Our Ideas are Confused
But our natural instincts, or common sense can also be affected by what we learn. What happens to most of us is that we start off on the wrong foot from the very beginning.

I was brought up on fried egg and chips and tomato sandwiches supplemented with enormous amounts of sweets and chocolates which I bought on the way to and from school (my mother now feeds herself very healthily but that happened well after I had left home.) Whatever you were fed on – whether it was 'meat and two veg', jam sandwiches, or fish and chips – if you can claim that you got off to a really healthy start, you'd hardly be reading this book. Those early learning patterns can last a lifetime, and distort our natural feeding habits from the start.

School hasn't set a very good example either. I used to love school meals, but looking back I can see that they were full of preserved meats (sausages and corned beef), cooked-to-death vegetables, and sugar. And if you had cookery lessons I'm willing to bet it was all the bad habits that were reinforced. 'Bring sugar, flour, butter, and cocoa tomorrow – we're going to be making chocolate cake.'

Some people ask their doctors what they think about diet. Most of them don't think very much about it at all. But that isn't the doctors' fault. Until very recently medical training included practically no information on diet beyond the basics, and the concept of healing with nutrition wasn't considered at all.

Now there's a new medical society in this country called the British Society for Nutritional Medicine,[3] which aims to put that right, but unless you're lucky enough to live near one of the two hundred or so members of the society, it will be years before you can go to your GP and expect him or her to 'think nutritionally'.

Books and Magazines

So where can we start to put matters right? Many people get their first ideas about nutrition from magazines. But magazines may contain anything from garbled rubbish to accurate reports on the state of the art. What most people forget is that these articles are written by journalists. And journalists are no more expert on the subjects about which they write than you are. They've mugged it up, sometimes by attending conferences and sometimes by reading other magazine articles, or by talking to one or two people on the phone.

This doesn't mean that there aren't any good nutritional journalists. But what they say is bound to be second or third hand because they are usually not involved in science or nutrition themselves. It can never be direct knowledge, no matter how authoritative it sounds, so you can never be sure how accurate it is.

Books on nutrition run the full spectrum too. Some are excellent, but many are quite whacky. Some are full of myths which are repeated by author after author without the truth of the matter ever being tested. And some contain ideas just coming in from the fringes of medicine and popular nutrition – usually ridiculed by the medical establishment and university nutritionists – but which one day may become the newly accepted dogma.

The fibre theory is a good example. Once regarded as a crazy idea, it's now promoted by leaflets in every doctor's waiting room, and there are hundreds of scientific papers written about it every year. The problem is that you have no way of knowing which crazy new idea is going to be tomorrow's sacred cow.

Fortunately there are some reliable books written for the general reader (see Recommended Reading page 251) some of which give accurate reports from nutritional research.

Don't Trust Only to Science
But if there's no way of knowing if you can trust what the popular books say, what about science? The problem

about science as a way of knowing is that it only investigates one piece of the truth at a time. When I am using science as a way to the truth I always remind myself about the blind men and the elephant.

It's an old Arab teaching story. Three blind old men were taken to an elephant and asked to say what they thought it was. One stumbled up and found the tail. 'Ah,' he said, 'it's a piece of old rope.' The next one came across one huge leg and said, 'This must be a tree.' The third caught the trunk and said, 'Good heavens, I'm being strangled by a snake.' Relying on *nothing but* science gives you no better chance of finding the real truth (the elephant) than the guesses of the blind old men.

With nutritional science you have to be doubly careful. Scientific research is very expensive, far too expensive these days for any ordinary university department to do it without outside funds. Even a small project could hardly get off the ground without at least a quarter of a million pounds. But the only wealthy institutions interested in sponsoring research into nutrition are – you've guessed it – the giant corporations of the food industry.

Ninety-nine per cent of the nutrition research in the world is sponsored by the big food companies. That doesn't mean of course that the research itself won't be genuine. But the emphasis of what is researched and what isn't, is obviously more influenced by what will make yet more money for the food manufacturers, than by what we as humans would like to know about feeding ourselves.

Trusting only to science to tell you how to feed yourself can never be fully satisfactory. It's like finding one piece of a jigsaw and having no idea where the other pieces are. Or how many there should be to make a whole picture. You can hardly postpone your next meal until all the pieces have been found. Nutrition is about feeding people, not ideas. We have to use a whole range of aproaches simultaneously when it's whole human beings we're learning to nourish.

The Wholistic Approach

I find I have four ways of getting to the bottom of what I want to understand, and putting all four together really helps me get a better view of whatever's going on.

The first way of course is science itself. I read the scientific reports and constantly refer to them when I'm trying to understand something. But because I think it's very important not to rely on science alone, I back that up with three other sources of information – observation of my clients and friends, research into the history of diet and the diet of other cultures, and finally what I can learn from my own body.

One of the oldest and most respected methods of gaining knowledge about healing is to observe people closely as they go through the healing process – a technique long used by herbalists and doctors. Nowadays it's given the name of 'clinical experience'.

Clinical Experience

I don't think my clients ever realise just how much they teach me. It's one thing to read a book about diseases of the digestive system, or the latest research into repopulating the gut with the correct bacteria. But it's altogether different to sit with someone with digestive difficulties and take in what they're saying, observe in detail how they're looking, and listen to how they say they feel. What's in front of you is not a case history nor an example from a book. He or she is a whole and unique human being.

Human beings have a funny way of not conforming to

textbook cases at all. When people first started consulting me, this worried me a great deal. I suffered from considerable concern because what my clients were telling me was frequently in complete contradiction to what the scientific literature described. Now I hope I've learned enough humility to realise that they're more likely to be right about their own experiences than I am (or the books).

Recently for instance I've been working with a woman who cannot sleep if she takes a supplement of zinc. If you read textbooks on mineral supplementation you'll find that the most likely effect of a large dose of zinc is that it will make you sleep.[4]

But not so with this client. When she takes a zinc supplement she can't sleep at all. Instead of brushing this inconsistency under the carpet as part of me would like to do, I believe her. I listen to everything she can tell me about it and I store it in my mind for future reference. One day I'll be listening to another client, or reading a new scientific report, and I'll suddenly know why that woman could not sleep when she took a zinc supplement. And that knowledge will help me with yet other unusual cases I may meet in the future.

You can do the same. I've never met anyone with an interest in nutrition who didn't have half a dozen stories to tell about friends and relatives and what nutritional strategies have helped them. These people are your teacher. Don't underestimate just how much you can learn from them (or they from you). Learn to take in what they're actually saying (rather than trying to fit them into some preconceived picture), and file it in your memory for future use. Doing this will teach you as much about your own health and nutrition as theirs.

Learning from History

The third way of 'knowing' I use is to look for knowledge from the past. Looking back at history can sometimes be a way of seeing the common sense of a thing very quickly.

Take, for instance, the continuing debate about just what quantity of vitamins and minerals we really need for health. Do you support the official view that a balanced diet supplies all the vitamins and minerals we need?[5] Or do you think the good old British diet is likely to leave us short, as other experts would have us believe?[6] Do you perhaps think it's dangerous to increase your vitamin and mineral intake, or do you believe it is advisable?

The official recommended daily intakes are worked out by averaging the diets and states of health of large groups of people.[7] But all that such an exercise can really tell us is how much of a vitamin we probably need to prevent a deficiency disease – like beri beri for instance which is caused by a deficiency of vitamin B1. The recommended daily intake doesn't take account of how much of a vitamin or mineral we might need for truly optimum health. It can't, because none of the groups of people used to work it out had anything like optimum health themselves.

That is why the argument about vitamins is never won. Neither side can really produce enough scientific evidence to prove or disprove their point of view, because there is no known community or group of people with a really high level of health whose diet can be studied in order to settle the matter.

But if we look into history we find some astonishingly good evidence that could actually settle the debate once and for all. In the 1920s an American dentist called Dr Weston A. Price made a remarkable contribution to our knowledge of the human diet.[8] Travelling the world at a time when there were still many populations living on traditional primitive diets, he was able to study and record what these people ate, and whether or not they were healthy. He went to remote Swiss valleys, to the islands of the Hebrides in Scotland, and he also visited the Eskimos, the Maoris, the Canadian Indians, the Australian Aborigines and many others.

Wherever he went he looked for a village or a community that was still eating the original diet of the region. And what he found was quite extraordinary. The level of health of every community still eating their so-called 'primitive' diet was far higher than was to be found in the so-called civilised Western world. Of course, healthy individuals are still to be found everywhere, but there are no longer whole communities with this overall high level of health. Today, although infectious diseases are largely under control, practically every degenerative disease is on the increase. But in the 1920s Weston Price was still able to find *whole villages with hardly a decayed tooth between them*. (Because he was a dentist Weston Price used the condition of the teeth and gums as a first monitor of health.)

So on the island of Taransay in the Hebrides, for instance, where the traditional diet was simply oatmeal porridge, oatcake and seafoods, he found less than one tooth in a hundred had ever been attacked by tooth decay. (If that happened in our society most dentists would be out of business.) And in spite of the apparently meagre diet, both adults and children of the island were outstandingly healthy, well built and strong.

Yet in the port of Stornoway on the nearby island of Lewis (where Weston Price found you could buy angel cake, white bread, jam, tinned vegetables, sweetened fruit juices and sweets of every kind) one in every four people actually had a whole mouth full of false teeth, and a new hospital had just been built to cope with the rapid progress of tuberculosis – a disease to which the Taransay islanders were apparently immune.

Wherever he travelled around the world Weston Price found the same thing – the communities living on their original diets (whatever their original diets were – they varied tremendously) had levels of health and freedom from disease practically unknown today. And just as certainly he found that wherever a community had made a change to the 'modern' Western diet, high in white flour and sugary foods, the level of health of that community had fallen precipitously within the lifetime of one generation.

Vitamins in the Primitive Diet

How does this knowledge help the vitamin debate? Fortunately for posterity Dr Weston Price actually analysed the diets of these people and left records of the amounts of vitamins and minerals they were eating.

These simple communities on their basic, and (by our standards) meagre, diets were actually consuming levels of vitamins and minerals far higher than we do today. In every case the level was higher than the present government recommended intake. The level of vitamin A for instance consumed daily by primitive communities all over the world (including the Eskimos, the Canadian Indians, the New Zealand Maoris, the Swiss, the Gaelics of the Hebrides and the Aborigines of Australia) was in excess of 50,000 international units. That is *at least ten times as high* as today's recommended daily intake!

So looking into historical records like these gives me a third perspective on diet and health. When I add this to what I have found in science, and what I have learned from my clients, I begin to grow a far more complete and reliable picture than trusting to science alone. As I develop each of these sources of knowledge I become more and more able to go to the root of the problems that I tackle, and solve them quickly. Almost invariably the answer is not one I could have got 'by the book'.

Listening to One's Body

But one of the most powerful and most neglected of all sources of knowledge is actually the body itself. Most people know someone (usually a granny) who feels things 'in her bones'. The very idea is almost a joke. Yet this is actually a remnant of an ancient and very powerful way of knowing. One that you must reawaken if you really want health and energy for your body.

One of the classic experiments of early psychology showed just how vital and reliable this 'body knowledge' can be, at least in small children. In a six-month study at the Mt Sinai Hospital, Cleveland, Ohio[9] in 1928, crawling babies were given complete freedom to choose from a selection of natural foods that were laid out before them, three times a day. It had never been suspected before that such young children would have any 'sense' about feeding themselves, but the results showed otherwise.

Although each of their tastes (and presumably needs) were somewhat different, each child actually gave itself a perfectly balanced diet using nothing but their own inborn sense. One child even cured his rickets over a period of four months by choosing extra cod liver oil and milk until he was healed. This inborn body knowledge is something with which nearly all of us have lost touch by the time we reach adulthood.

But it can be rekindled. People phone me and say, 'I've

got this hankering to eat liver, but the books say meat is bad for me. What do you think?' My answer is always to forget the books and listen to your body. The more you do, the more you'll get to know and trust the signals it gives you and as time goes on your confidence will grow. It's rather like learning to swim. It comes in fits and starts at first, and you have to go under a few times before you start to get the hang of it.

But once your body knowledge is alive again you'll have the answer to so much of what you've been wanting to know. Then your body will be a better guide to what you need than the instructions of a nutritionist or the edicts of any diet book. For this natural body knowledge is none other than the lost instinct – the instinct that I hope, with the help of the Wright Diet, you will learn to use again.

Reawakening The Lost Instinct

What happened to me was that my natural body instinct gradually grew stronger over the years (as I was developing the Wright Diet). But one particular incident really let me know how far I had come. Until a few years ago I was a regular wine drinker. I suppose I drank an average of a bottle a week, often taking a glass in the evening. Then one summer I developed a tooth abscess and decided to take a fruit fast to clear it. By the end of ten days the abscess had gone and I was feeling fantastic. With the heightened sensitivity that often comes with such a cleansing I went slowly back on to the Wright Diet and found that among the various foods and drinks I didn't at first feel attracted to was wine.

I thought nothing of it at first; it's quite common to feel choosy about what you eat and drink after a fast. But several weeks later when we were taking a brief summer break at a hotel in Devon, Brian asked me if I would share a bottle of wine with him, and without thinking (or checking with my body) I said I would. Fortunately I took the precaution of ordering a bottle of Perrier water along with Brian's choice of wine. It was lucky that I did. Because I couldn't lift that wine to my mouth all evening. Each time I tried my stomach said, 'not right now, I'll have some in a minute' and my hand swerved to the Perrier. When I finally did take a determined swig at the wine, my throat simply refused to swallow.

That was the first time I really experienced that my body 'knew' better than my head. I doubt if I've drunk as much as a bottle of wine in all the years since then, not because I've tried to stop myself, but because that experience of my body just not wanting it has stayed with me. I have since discovered that I actually have an intolerance of grapes and therefore of wine – something my body obviously knew instinctively long before I worked it out using my head.

Instinct Comes Naturally on the Wright Diet

In fact there's nothing mysterious about body knowledge and the way to reawaken it. You can start by looking at the food that you're about to eat and then tuning into or 'feeling' your stomach (just below your bottom ribs) and asking your stomach how it feels about each item on your plate. You'll soon begin to get a message back – 'oh no, please, not cheese again, it hurts my lining' or 'mmm, rice, how delicious' or 'fish? well OK'.

This rekindling of a direct and essential relationship with your body actually comes very easily on the Wright Diet. You don't have to try. One of the first signs that the diet is working is the increased consciousness that it brings. People say, 'my body's feeling so different' or 'I can feel my kidneys for the first time' or 'I'm getting a real appetite for all those salads – I can feel what they're doing for me', and you know that a process of awakening has started that will continue month after month as the diet gently does its work. On the Wright Diet you'll find you can stop asking all those questions, because your body itself will be telling you the answers.

3
The Wright Direction

Once you've understood the principles that lie behind the Wright Diet you could virtually work out the diet for yourself. And that's just how it should be. What's the use of books that tell you how you should eat without giving any good reason, as though the whole thing just came down the mountain with Moses along with the Ten Commandments?

Every one of the principles given below has been tested in each of the four ways I've outlined in Chapter 2. They're all backed up with sound scientific data; they've been shown to bring significant increases in health to a large number of people; they have their roots in history and the way we've always fed our bodies; and they 'feel' right – to me and my clients.

The Wright Diet will give you the opportunity to test each one of them for yourself. Some will give you more benefits than others since we all have slightly different needs from each other. Indeed, that is one of the main principles of the Wright Diet.

Correct Your Acid/Alkaline Balance

You can spend a lifetime trying to get to the bottom of your problems: psychotherapy, astrology, Harley Street doctors – the list is endless. Yet I sometimes wonder if this simple principle of diet hasn't got as much to offer as the best of them. Get your acid/alkaline balance right and a lot of other things in your life will fall into place.

As a child I used to chant the poem of *Bad Sir Botany* by A. A. Milne.[1] 'Sir Brian had a battleaxe with great big knobs on; he went among the villagers and blipped them on the head!' It used to give me enormous pleasure – I knew just how he felt! I had a feeling of wanting to rage at the world too. And that feeling stayed with me as I grew up. I got over wanting to blip people on the head, of course, but I was still aware of a seething just below the surface, an irritation that could easily be scratched, a quality of frustration and anger.

Little did I suspect that a feeling like that could stem from anything so absurdly simple as the acid/alkaline balance of my blood. Yet when Marshall Lever (my first nutrition guide) put me on a high alkaline diet, something important in my life did change – I began to feel more at home on this planet.

Alkalinity Feels Good

When people talk about acid/alkaline balance they're talking about the alkalinity of the blood. The blood is naturally slightly alkaline. (It has an average pH of 7.4.) But it can vary enough to make the difference between feeling good and calm, or more like a cross rat that just fell out the wrong side of bed. Fortunately the variation is not wide. If the pH strayed too far either way our health would be at serious risk. But the body actually takes very good care to maintain the balance, using several different mechanisms to 'buffer' the changes in the blood.

By breathing out more carbon dioxide for example, we can alkalise the blood. That's why deep breathing can make us feel so good. Many Eastern breathing exercises are working on precisely this principle. The body can also keep the pH of the blood in balance by controlling how much acid is pushed out through the urine, and by drawing on alkaline reserves that can be used to neutralise excess acidity.

Changing Your Acid/Alkaline Balance

But day by day there's one vital way we have of influencing the alkalinity of our blood. And that's the food that we eat. We can feel clear and strong and relaxed after eating, or we can feel as irritable as that rat. What makes the difference is the balance between acid- and alkaline-forming foods that a meal contains.

Most of us eat 95 per cent acid-forming foods at every meal of our life. Toast and marmalade, coffee and sugar for instance is an all acid-forming breakfast. A hamburger, bun and french fries are almost entirely acid-forming too.

Potatoes are actually alkaline-forming, as are most other vegetables, but their alkaline-forming qualities come from the minerals they contain, and these are mostly lost in the cooking water or neutralised by the acidity of frying oils. Potatoes (whichever way they're cooked), vegetables, and the odd glass of orange juice are practically the only alkaline-forming foods that most of us ever eat. Full details of which foods are acid- and which are alkaline-forming are given on page 224, but here is a rough working guide:

Acid-Forming	Alkaline-Forming
Meat	Most vegetables
Poultry	Most fruits
Fish	Some nuts
Eggs	Milk
Grains	
Some nuts	
Cheese	

You may be surprised to find that orange juice (the real thing, that is) is alkaline-forming. So indeed are lemons, grapefruit, and limes. When you taste the juice of these fruits they're acid, of course. Your mouth knows that instinctively. But when they, or any other food, are digested by the body they're broken down until all that remains is an 'ash' in the bloodstream (just like the remains of last night's fire). And all citrus fruit, when completely digested, give an alkaline ash.)

What actually determines whether a food is acid- or alkaline-forming is the mineral content of this ash. If it's high in calcium, magnesium, sodium or potassium then the food which produced it is alkaline-forming:[2] it will contribute to the alkaline reserves of the body. When the minerals phosphorus, sulphur and chlorine predominate, on the other hand, the food is said to be acid-forming:[2] it will reduce the alkalinity of the blood and force the body to draw on its alkaline reserves.

The food that most of us eat is roughly 90–95 per cent acid-forming whereas the ideal is probably more like 60–80 per cent the other way. Eating up to 80 per cent alkaline-forming foods should provide you with optimum alkalinity for your blood and tissues. Although the modern diet is so acid, there are good historical reasons for thinking that the alkaline diet is actually more natural.

Our Ancestors Ate an Alkaline Diet
Before the day that someone saved a few ears of grain and realised that you could grow more if you planted it (this happened first about ten thousand years ago), we all made our living by hunting and food gathering. Judging by historical research (but also by observation because there are still a few hunter-gatherer peoples living today[3]), the hunters would go hunting daily, and the women and

the children would go out gathering whatever berries and edible roots and shoots they could find. The meat that the hunters brought home was acid-forming of course. But modern studies of hunter-gatherers have shown that the hunters are only successful about a quarter of the time.[4] So meat forms between 25 and 33 per cent of their diet. The rest of their food, gathered by the women, is from plant sources and therefore almost entirely alkaline-forming.

Experts who have studied hunter-gatherers consider that it was the most successful and persistent adaptation man has ever achieved and that 'the biology of our species was created in that long gathering and hunting period'.[5] If this is the case then the balance of the hunter-gatherers' diet could be a key for us. The hunter-gatherers ate a 60–70 per cent alkaline-forming diet.

The Alkaline Experience
The most immediate experience of turning your diet around in this way and eating up to 80 per cent alkaline-forming foods is one of overwhelming well-being, calmness, emotional stability, strength without aggression, a feeling of constant optimism. It's only when you have your blood at that upper alkaline limit that you begin to appreciate that the body and the mind really are one. When you feel good, you feel very very good, good in body, good in mind.

The state of acidosis on the other hand is like a mirror image. You feel as though you've got a constant hangover: grouchy, sensitive, exhausted; inclined to aches and pains, headaches and sleeplessness; probably with a sour stomach and acid sweat (which might even be sufficient to damage silk close to the skin, or to discolour jewellery).

Psychiatrists and sociologists are going to have to start taking note of this vital dietary factor. The American criminologist Alexander Schauss already considers the acid-alkaline balance of diet an important factor when working with delinquents and criminals.[6] Even cravings and addictions respond to increased alkalinity. Dr Stanley Schachter and colleagues of the Department of Psychology at New York's Columbia University showed that people actually smoke more cigarettes when their urine is acid.[7] So the Wright Diet will actually help you to stop smoking, reduce your cravings, and give you back your freedom of choice.

But what really matters is your own experience. There would be no point in changing the acid/alkaline balance of your diet if it didn't work for you. Try it. The Wright Diet will show you how. I've never known anybody, once they'd tried it for a fortnight, who didn't want to go on. Of course you'll fall off the wagon now and then, but the marvellous way you feel on a high alkaline intake will pull you back to it again and again.

Balance Your Blood Sugar

Knowing where your energy comes from is probably more important than having money, a car, or even a job. The real achievers out there in this world are the ones who have the unlimited energy, the balance and the staying power. People who are too tired to 'get it together', who are up one day and down the next, or who don't seem to have the energy to even care, are unlikely to achieve their simplest dreams. If this sounds too much like you, you can change. Learning how to recover your energy supply is surprisingly simple.

Have you ever asked yourself how long you could go without eating or drinking one of these: coffee, tea, alcohol, soft drinks, sweets, chocolate, ice cream, biscuits, pastries, cakes or good old-fashioned bread and jam? Can you, for instance, go for one whole day without any of them, without going weak at the knees? If you can I congratulate you. For these apparently innocent little items of twentieth-century diet have become the major fuels on which most people run their lives. In fact the vast majority of the human race now seems to need sugar, caffeine or alcohol at regular intervals just to get them through the day.

But the main essential of a fuel, surely, is that it should work? And sugar, especially glucose sugar, does work, doesn't it? All athletes know that. Caffeine too is certainly a pick-me-up. You feel that whenever you drink it. And anyone who has ever turned to alcohol for a spot of dutch courage has likewise felt the strength of whisky in their veins. But the trouble with all these energy sources is that they're a bit like doing a car journey with the choke out – you run along in overdrive for a while, then the fuel runs out.

And this is the problem. None of these stimulants or quick energy inputs can keep you going for very long. So you have to keep coming back for more. As long as you do that, you can keep going. Or at least stagger from one emergency snack to the next. But one of the drawbacks of using instant fuels like these is that you start to lose your instinct for the fuels the human body was really designed for – first class proteins such as fish, eggs, and meat; and complex carbohydrates like grains, pulses and root vegetables – and come to rely instead on a series of sugar and caffeine injections at regular intervals throughout the day.

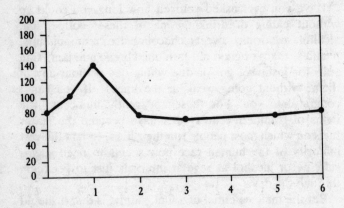

1 Normal
The blood sugar curve of a healthy individual. At no time during the six hours does the blood sugar fall much below the fasting level (the first reading).

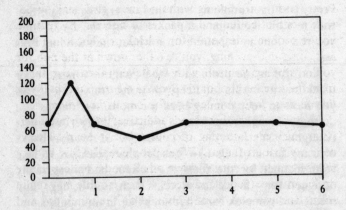

2 Mild Pre-Hypoglycemia
The speed of descent of the curve suggests rapid insulin reaction to the sugar stimulus.

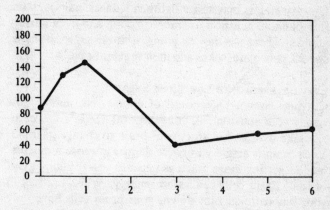

3 Reactive Hypoglycemia
The blood sugar drops below the fasting level within two hours of eating sugar.

One Thing Leads to Another

Pretty soon you're going without lunch, and 'making do' with a cup of coffee and a packet of biscuits. By teatime you're probably desperate for a drink or a chocolate bar, and come mid-evening, you're either down at the pub, or you're stuffing yourself with whatever takes your fancy from the kitchen cupboard. *Because the truth is that if you live on these fuels you can't go for long without them.*

And not only are these foods addictive, they're fattening. (Caffeine isn't fattening of course but it nearly always comes with lots of sugar.) When people realise this, and try to lose weight by cutting down on all foods, but especially on sugar, sweet foods and alcohol, then trouble may really start. Because once you're hooked on the quick ups and downs of energy that these fast foods can give you, you can't just cut them out (unless you know how) without suffering cravings, and even withdrawal symptoms.

Unwary dieters may suffer lightheadedness, nausea, pain, trembling, exhaustion, memory fogging and even anxiety attacks – because they're going without sugar, biscuits, sweets, chocolate, cakes and their regular tipple!

Cravings Come with Low Blood Sugar

Cravings cannot be ignored of course. No matter how strong your self-control, your physical needs will eventually take over and instruct your brain to change its mind. Your brain is actually in grave danger at those moments. You're getting those cravings because you're running out of fuel. Brain cells can't store energy. When the fuel in your bloodstream runs down, your brain cells have only one choice – get a new source of energy quickly, or start to die . . . you reach for the chocolate bar, the biscuits, the cream bun or the whisky . . . and that can be the start of a binge.

Sugar, caffeine and alcohol (and other foods, not to mention cigarettes) give us energy by doing just one thing – they help raise the level of glucose in our bloodstream. Glucose, or 'blood sugar' as it's often called, is the actual fuel that our bodies use. Cars run on petrol, we run on glucose. No matter what foods we eat, they can't give us a drop of energy until they've been broken down into glucose. This is why glucose itself can give us such instant energy. And since anything made from ordinary sugar (sucrose) is quickly converted into glucose, all those sweets, desserts and sugary snack foods give us rapid energy too.

The caffeine in coffee, tea, chocolate and cola drinks has the same effect by a slightly different route. Caffeine probably works by stimulating your adrenal glands (see the next chapter) to produce hormones that raise your blood sugar. Many other substances can do this too, among them salt and salty foods, nicotine and some food additives. In fact stress of any kind raises blood sugar, which is why you can get so hooked on it. Even getting scared watching a horror movie can raise your blood sugar.

So when it's instant energy we're after either one of these food types – the concentrated calories (sugar etc.), or the stimulants (caffeine, salt and so on) will do the trick. The trouble is, they give us rapid energy all right, but it's the kind that's going to run out again all too soon. For most people on a sugar/caffeine addiction cycle, this time interval may be down to one or two hours, or even less. This means you're going to run out of energy and get hungry again five or ten times a day (some people even wake up in the night with this problem).

But why should these concentrated sources of energy such as sugar only give us fuel for so short a time? Surely we don't use up all those condensed calories so quickly? Indeed we don't. Understanding that is part of the secret we should all know if we want to start using our energy wisely. When we eat high sugar foods, the level of glucose in our bloodstream surges rapidly. For a time we feel marvellous, full of go, ready to get on with the job. Children respond quickly too, usually by hurtling round the house like jet trains, their voices at maximum pitch and their feet hardly touching the floor. But uncontrolled blood glucose is a danger to the brain. It can't be allowed to rise too far. A body that doesn't take steps to bring that level down is suffering from diabetes.

A healthy body actually takes action the moment the sugar hits the taste buds. As soon as the message comes down the line that an attack of sugar is on its way the pancreas (see the next chapter) begins to pump out the hormone insulin. So, as fast as the sugar is pouring into the bloodstream, your pancreas is frantically pulling it out again and storing it (as glycogen) in your muscles and liver. Whatever's left over when the glycogen stores have been filled, *fatties please note*, is converted into fat and stored in your fat cells.

Do You Have Hypoglycemia?

The faster blood sugar goes up, the faster it's likely to come down. The fact is our bodies weren't designed to handle such concentrated fuels. Five hundred years ago most of us wouldn't have tasted sugar in our whole lifetime. Now we consume an average of 90 lbs each every year. Assaulting our bodies like that year after year can lead to over-sensitive reactions. In a condition that's sometimes called 'trigger happy' pancreas, the amount of insulin secreted doesn't just bring the level back to normal – it overshoots, and can leave us with less glucose in our bloodstream than when we started.

Recently scientists have shown that when we eat high sugar foods the muscles and tissues of the body become much more sensitive (in fact eleven times more sensitive) to the hormone insulin.[8] What this means is that whenever we eat a significant amount of sugar, our tissues, triggered by the insulin, start to pull glucose out of our bloodstream eleven times as fast as usual. This can leave us with low blood sugar and a raging appetite in a short space of time.

Medical opinion differs as to how many people suffer from the condition known as hypoglycemia (or low blood sugar). In this country it's thought to be fairly rare. But in America it's much more widely recognised. When 238 obese patients were given the glucose tolerance test at the Hahnemann Hospital in Philadelphia, 101 were diagnosed as hypoglycemic[9] (that's 42 per cent). When United Airlines tested 177 pilots, 44 had it[10] (that's 25 per cent).

And in a survey of 42,000 households conducted by the US Department of Health, Education and Welfare some 66,000 people reported having the condition[11] (almost one out of two).

One physician, Dr Sam E. Roberts, wrote in his book *Exhaustion, causes and treatment:* 'Hypoglycemia is probably the most common disease in the United States . . . I would estimate that at least fifty percent of the work in this country is done by people who are extremely tired or exhausted – and don't know it. Often they do not mention fatigue or exhaustion as a chief complaint. They have accepted it as part of life!'

This closely matches our seven years' experience at the Green Farm Nutrition Centre, except if anything I would put the figure rather higher than one in two. If, like the vast majority of us, you've grown up on a high sugar diet, I don't think it's so much a question of whether or not you have hypoglycemia, but rather *just how badly or how mildly you have it*. But 'having hypoglycemia' isn't like having tuberculosis or bunions. Hypoglycemia is only a fancy name for an adaptation your body has made to deal with your twentieth-century diet. Hypoglycemia can be cured. I'm an ex-hypoglycemic myself.

High Energy on the Wright Diet

The Wright Diet starts this process by putting you back on all those good old-fashioned fuels for which your body was built: the proteins and the complex carbohydrates. That means eating fish, meat, eggs, nuts, whole grains (rice, wheat, oats) or pulses (such as beans and lentils) at sufficient intervals through the day. Some authorities recommend only the protein foods for low blood sugar.[12] But we find that the complex carbohydrates are more natural and effective, avoiding the dangers of a high protein diet. For most people a combination of the two is ideal.

The timing of your meals is as important as what's in them. You have to eat often enough to prevent your blood sugar from falling. Getting to know how often you need to eat is one of the keys to success. At the beginning this may be every two hours. That's why the Wright Diet caters for morning and afternoon snacks. A well-timed mid-meal snack can save you from countless crises. Once you've got that rhythm of feeding yourself the foods you really need, you'll be able to cut out the biscuits, the sweets and the fancy puddings without any problem. You'll be able to cut down on coffee and tea as well. In fact the Wright Diet can help you get over much more than a sugar or a caffeine addiction. It can help you give up smoking or get over a drinking problem too.

Once the high sugar foods are out of your life you'll lose excess weight of course. (This is just one of the ways the Wright Diet works for weight loss, see Part Two.) But the really big changes will come in the way you feel. On the Wright Diet you'll find energy you haven't felt since you were a child. The diet will help you find inner strength too – the ability to make decisions for instance (and carry them through). But the best news is that you're going to feel so good, so balanced. Because your blood sugar needs are met with ease on the Wright Diet, all those day-to-day feelings of irritation and anxiety will vanish. Even depression may soon be a thing of the past.

Eat Organically Grown Food When You Can

Finding the odd slug on the cabbage when I'm making salad these days does the strangest things to me. It takes me straight back to childhood – and reminds me of a time when the world seemed full of fresh air and all things green and good. When I was a child I was squeamish. These days I don't mind those little slugs at all. When I find them I know that the food I'm about to eat is real – organically grown and free from pesticides and other chemicals.

For the last forty years or so we've all been taking part in an experiment with our food. It's probably the biggest change in our diets since that first clever idiot worked out how to take the bran and wheatgerm out of the flour. This recent experiment then, has been to use chemicals (which are totally foreign to the human body) to boost the growth rate, 'shelf life' and profitability of our food – using artificial fertilisers, pesticides, fungicides and so on. *It is now time for us to admit that the experiment has failed.*

The vast problems created by this experiment first came to notice when a book called *Silent Spring* by Rachel Carson was published in 1962.[13] The message of the book was clear. DDT, one of the early insecticides, had been discovered in 1939 – in time to be used extensively in the Second World War. By 1962 hundreds of millions of pounds of DDT had been released around the world and it was estimated that it had already saved 500 million lives – from malaria, typhus and other infectious diseases. But the price of all this was that DDT was by then on every surface of the planet, and in the body of every living creature. And there was growing evidence that the long-term effect of even this low level exposure might lead to serious health risks such as cancer.

The Extent of the Problem
DDT has since been banned (although it is still found on fruit and vegetables in this country[14]), but other

potentially harmful chemicals have taken its place. The blacklist of the Pesticides Action Network,[15] who are now campaigning for stricter government control, names chemicals such as Aldrin, 2,4,5-T, Captan and Dichlorvos all in regular use in this country, and some even sold for home gardening, which are known or suspected to cause birth defects, spontaneous abortion, genetic changes and cancer.[16]

Agricultural chemicals such as these are now found not only in the fruit and vegetables we buy, but in the flour, the bread, the meat and therefore in virtually all canned, frozen and packeted goods (unless of course they specifically claim to have been organically grown). According to the Ministry of Agriculture's own estimates only 1 per cent of vegetables grown for human consumption are not treated with pesticides. Most potato, onion and cabbage crops receive up to 10 doses. In 1982, one crop of lettuce was reported to have been sprayed 46 times, with four different chemicals being used.

There is concern too about the increasing use of artificial fertilisers. The chemical nitrate, on which these fertilisers are based, is washed into the streams and reservoirs and thence into our drinking water. It gets into our fruit and vegetables too. In itself nitrate is fairly harmless, but it can be transformed within the body into its nastier relative, nitrite. Nitrites may then combine in the stomach with amino acids (from the proteins in our food) to form nitrosamines[17] – chemicals that are known to cause cancer, and are now also thought to be a cause of juvenile onset diabetes.[18] (Nitrites are actually added to almost all preserved meats, such as bacon and sausages, to prevent botulism and keep their colour pink.)

Once you start looking at this kind of information it's all too easy to get overwhelmed. Don't. We've been developing the power to risk our health in this way for over forty years, but at the same time we've been acquiring the nutritional knowledge of how to heal and defend ourselves more effectively. You can help protect yourself from the harmful effects of nitrites and the other chemicals by getting enough vitamin C and other nutrients (see page 231 for the supplement guidelines).

It's obvious at the same time that we should be eating organically grown, unsprayed foods whenever we can. Have a look at the Useful Addresses page 244 for details of the Organic Food Guide which will help you to find what's available in your area. BUT, and this is a very big but, *you must eat the regular sprayed ones when you can't find chemical-free vegetables.* Don't go without, especially not without vegetables, because you can't find the unsprayed ones. Whatever proportion of organic foods and vegetables you can bring into the Wright Diet will be helping you work towards your long-term health. Beyond that stop worrying. Or the worry will do you more harm than the chemicals.

Meat and Dairy Foods are Affected Too

One day in 1949 an American scientist working with the latest wonder drug, the antibiotic tetracycline, made a discovery that was to change the course of animal farming, perhaps for ever. The researcher, Dr Thomas Jukes, wasn't exactly interested in the antibiotic. He was looking for something that would produce significant amounts of vitamin B12 (then a rare commodity), because he had a theory that the vitamin could boost the growth rate of livestock animals. Finding relatively high concentrations in the left-overs of the process that produced the antibiotic, Jukes and his colleagues decided to give some of this left-over mash to baby chicks to see what would happen.

Even now, nearly forty years later, few people are aware of the full significance of what did happen in that experiment. The chicks made weight gains of between 10 per cent and 20 per cent above normal;[19] these were growth increases previously unheard of. When Jukes and his colleagues tried the mash on pigs it worked even better. But to their astonishment it wasn't the vitamin in the mash that was pushing up the animals' growth rate, *it was the antibiotic*.

Just how antibiotics promote growth in animals is still an unsolved question, but for the last thirty years antibiotics have been added to the feed of practically all livestock animals both in this country and in America – a practice that has changed the face of animal farming beyond all recognition. Not only has it given farmers a vast increase in profits, it has also meant that animals could be crowded into confined spaces as never before, without risk of disease – intensive farming in fact, with the appalling change of lifestyle that this has meant for the animals involved. But for us humans it has meant a far reaching change too, and one that is potentially every bit as health-threatening. *That change is that we now get a dose of antibiotic in virtually every bite of meat, eggs and dairy foods that we eat.*

What are the Consequences?

This low level exposure to antibiotics can have far reaching effects. Anyone who's ever taken a course of antibiotics to fight infection knows what the side effects can be: problems with digestion such as bloating, wind, constipation or diarrhoea, and increased sensitivity to foods. Post-antibiotic depression is fairly common too, and there can be temporary loss of hair in the weeks following treatment. Now this is what can happen when we take a full dose of antibiotic. What shows up with low level exposure is more subtle, but in the long term just as devastating.

Most of the side effects come from the destruction of the natural bacteria of the colon. Because, of course, antibiotics don't only destroy the bacteria causing infection, they also wipe out the good guys – the intestinal flora. The intestine is actually a human garden. And the helpful bacteria that live there are its flowers – that's why they're called the 'flora' (see the next chapter). Not only do the flora help with digestion, they're known to be naturally antibiotic and anti-tumour too.[20] Imagine what would happen if you poured a can of herbicide over your garden every day. Some weeds would die, yes, but so would most of the flowers. Soon only the resistant species would survive.

This is just what happens in our intestines. Those daily doses of antibiotics knock out most of the bacteria we need for digestion and good health. This leaves the field wide open for the resistant and more destructive bacteria (such as salmonella[21]) to take over. It also allows yeast organisms such as *Candida Albicans* to thrive[22] and this can trigger an increased sensitivity to foods, and sometimes a wide-scale disruption of our health.[23] For most of us though, because of the loss of a healthy flora, this continuous exposure to antibiotic drugs simply means a lowered ability to digest and handle our food, and possibly a lowered resistance to gut infections and other imbalances such as cancer.

Hormones in Your Beef
There are other growth promoters in meats too. Hormones, no longer permitted to be put into animal feeds,

are now given as ear implants. One variety in particular worries Dr Schoental of the Department of Pathology at the Royal Veterinary College.[24] The hormone used, called zeranol, is a form of the female hormone oestrogen which is derived from the mould *fusarium*. What concerns Dr Schoental is that this mould also commonly occurs on crops harvested in damp weather, so that the level of natural oestrogens in our food can sometimes be quite high.

High levels of oestrogens are known to promote cancers of the breast, prostate, endometrium and ovary (and also possibly of the thyroid, testes and bone[25]). This means that women on the pill, pregnant women (whose children may be affected), and men too can be vulnerable to an overload of oestrogens in our diet. The oestrogens we get from beef, although not high in themselves, may in certain circumstances, Dr Schoental believes, be the straw that breaks the camel's back.

Many other growth promoters and drugs are in common use on today's farms, among them copper-containing formulas which threaten to shift the balance of zinc and other minerals in our body. Government regulations stipulate that many of these drugs must be withdrawn several days before the animals go to slaughter. But there is no enforcement of this rule, and many of the informed sources that I spoke to had serious doubts that many farmers actually do this.

It often isn't possible to stop eating factory farmed meat and dairy products just like that. Nor should you worry unduly. These foods aren't poisonous; it's just a question of degree. In the short term your body can probably handle the antibiotics and growth promoters. But if it's optimum well-being that you're seeking (as well as your long-term health) I believe that you need to look for better quality food.

The Wright Diet encourages you to look around and see what's available in your area. Fortunately there are now farmers, animal feed producers, butchers and shop-keepers who want to offer meat and dairy products free of drugs. At least one good butcher offers a nationwide meat delivery service (see Useful Addresses page 244), and organic, or additive-free dairy produce is available in many health shops and at farm doors in many parts of the country. The more we use these services the more we encourage them. Additive-free meat, milk, eggs and cheese cost a little more, but what sense does it make to count costs when it's your health that you're dealing with?

Eat At Least Half Your Food Raw

If you've never made your own salad of succulent, raw vegetables – fine slices of fresh-from-the-garden cabbage, covered by sweet, grated carrots and beetroot, crunchy chunks of celery, soft slices of avocado, a few piquant stems of spring onion, and two or three whole baby tomatoes (the kind that really smell like tomatoes), dressed with virgin olive oil, fresh lemon and herbs – then you have never experienced the full possibility of raw foods. The old lettuce-tomato-and-cucumber routine simply will not serve as the token to raw foods in your life.

There are several good scientific reasons why raw foods can do so much for your health, but the most powerful incentive is quite simply *the experience*. For ourselves, from the moment we started, it felt marvellous to be going shopping for really healthy vegetables rather than the lifeless kind that most people put up with. Washing and then chopping them on a wooden board, taking in the sweet and sharp smells, and making a delicious dressing – all this has been part of the ritual of our lives for the last ten years. What we find most remarkable is how dreadful you feel, once you've started this routine, if you have to go without your raw foods for more than a day at a time. Raw foods add a quality to your life that just can't yet be fully explained by science.

Raw fruits and vegetables are packed with vitamins and minerals of course, and many of these are lost or destroyed when you cook them. Three quarters of the vitamin C is lost outright, and a good proportion of the B vitamins too.[26] The water you drain from these cooked vegetables is full of magnesium and potassium, two truly vital minerals which we need for calming nerves and relaxing muscles. Indeed it's largely because fresh vegetables are so packed with these minerals that they have such power to alkalise and re-energise the body.

Enzyme Power
Another bonus is the natural enzyme content of both fruit and vegetables before they are cooked.[27] Every living cell contains the enzymes it needs to digest itself.[28] Eating plant foods in their raw state allows the body to take full advantage of these enzymes during digestion, reducing the need for the stomach and pancreas to produce so much of their own. This takes a huge burden off the digestion, and leads to a feeling of lightness and clarity, so different from the heavy stodgy feeling we have when we eat most cooked dinners. Cooking your food on the other hand completely destroys these enzymes.

Until recently it was doubted that the enzymes in plant

foods could actually help us with digestion, because scientists assumed that the enzymes would be broken down by the stomach making them useless. Now there is growing evidence to the contrary[29] – that plant enzymes can indeed aid digestion. Many African nations have always known this. In these countries the traditional ending to a meal is paw-paw or papaya, a fruit densely packed with the enzyme papain, capable of digesting up to one hundred times its own weight of the toughest protein.

But it isn't only digestion that benefits from eating in this way. Raw plant foods, because of their powerful alkalising properties and their high mineral content, have a power to lift our mood. Nothing shifts depression so fast as living on nothing but raw fruit and vegetables for a few days (see Part Two). Ultimately, however, it is the overriding quality of well-being that becomes so addictive to raw food eaters. Once you have tasted that quality in your life you'll find it hard to go without.

Foods that Shouldn't be Eaten Raw

There are some provisos however. Raw food eating really refers to vegetables and fruit. Animal foods should not be eaten raw (Japanese raw fish dishes are an exception, but they need to be extremely fresh). Raw eggs contain avidin, a protein which destroys the B vitamin biotin in the body (and is neutralised by light cooking). And raw meat and eggs both contain trypsin inhibitors (trypsin is one of our body's protein digesting enzymes), which makes them difficult to digest in the raw state.

Many members of the bean family also contain trypsin inhibitors, and some contain actual poisons (red kidney beans for instance) which are eliminated with adequate cooking. Nearly all pulses (peas, beans and lentils) should be cooked, and some, such as red kidney and soya beans, for several hours. In some cases sprouting (see the Sprouting Guide page 190) also gets rid of these negative factors, allowing us to eat beanshoots and other pulses in their raw state.

There are also grains which can be eaten uncooked – raw wheatgerm and muesli for instance – but they should be soaked, preferably overnight, for optimum digestibility.[29] Some people however can't handle raw grains (see Chapter 6 for guidance). If your stomach goes on strike when it sees oat and wheat flakes floating amongst the nuts, milk and raisins, you could be one of these. If so don't eat them. Cook your oats and other grains in the good old-fashioned way (see recipes).

Let's Not Forget the Balance

In our enthusiasm for eating all good things raw, we shouldn't lose sight of the tremendous push forward that cooking has given to humanity. Cooking has probably been at least as responsible for the great leap forward as the discovery of the wheel and the adoption of grains. No creature on earth has such a wide and varied diet as man. That we have been able to pick our foods from amongst this incredible variety (considering how narrow is the range of most other species' foods) has largely been due to our discovery of cooking, which makes many otherwise indigestible foods available to us.

The health food dogma that raw is always best is nonsense. In fact raw food eating has little historical precedent. There's no evidence that the primitive people that Weston Price and other early explorers visited, ever ate their food raw. The same is true of third world villages today. The explorer Christina Dodwell wrote to me recently, 'Raw foods (except fruit) are seldom eaten by third world villagers. One reason is that most of their staple foods need extensive cooking to make them tender. Green vegetable soup is the commonest dish.

'Another reason for not eating raw foods is because the water is not always very pure, and plain washed vegetables can be the cause of sickness. One piece of advice I'd give to travellers is to avoid eating salads (it's surprising how often they cause diarrhoea) unless you wash them yourself in boiled water. Even so, in countries like China where human faeces are used as fertilisers it's safer to cook food properly. The difference is that in the third world one is trying to avoid bugs and sickness, which is not a problem in England.[30]'

This doesn't mean of course that there's anything wrong in us taking our food raw. On the contrary raw foods can give us benefits that our ancestors (and third world cousins) never suspected. It's really a question of balance. If you live in a country where the water and the vegetables are not contaminated, then you have the opportunity to test for yourself what eating raw fruit and vegetables can do for you. The Wright Diet will show you how. After a couple of weeks I doubt that you'll ever want to give up eating some of your foods raw.

Cook Simply

There's a world of difference between a simply-cooked and nourishing meal (served with a large raw vegetable salad), and the kind of cooked-to-death dishes that most of us live on. Cooking may kill off the bugs and the natural poisons – but if we're not careful it could kill us too. For, in the long term, some of our everyday cooking techniques may cause birth defects, cellular changes and cancer.

Boiling vegetables and pouring the water down the sink may not be exactly life-threatening, but those continued losses of vital minerals will eventually undermine your health. Steaming vegetables on the other hand (if you must cook them) leads to minimal losses and delicious eating. This is the kind of change you need to make in your cooking habits, if you want to reach high level health and feel like a full human being again.

Cooking meals that are healthy is very simple. You need little equipment and even less time. When we had a new kitchen fitted in our house we were looking for a simple and nourishing space in which to prepare our daily meals. The last thing we wanted was a mass of sophisticated double ovens, rotisseries and microwave equipment. We ended up with one good oven of the old-fashioned variety, four burners (though we rarely use more than one or two), a fridge, a freezer, a food processor, a baking tray and three saucepans.

When we cook it's done simply. We bake fish with herbs in a little water. We boil pulses, except for falafels which we bake without oil instead of deep frying (see the recipes). We simmer soups and stews in the winter. For parties we might bake a simple cake or biscuits. Occasionally we steam a vegetable. We don't cook puddings. We don't fry. The real focus in our kitchen is on *not cooking*.

We prepare our food in this way because it feels and tastes so good. Food that is lightly cooked, and free of oxidised oils and fats (which happens when you cook with oil), gives you an experience of eating that reminds you of what feeling good is all about. Food prepared in this way is digestible. It doesn't sit on your stomach, or leave you gripping your liver. Most of us expect discomfort after eating as a matter of course. On the Wright Diet this will be a thing of the past.

Cooking Can be Dangerous

We have some very sound reasons for cooking as simply as we do. The art of healthy cooking is to get the benefits – increased digestibility and freedom from bugs and other bothers – without incurring the disadvantages. And these can be considerable: Japanese researchers have shown for instance that protein foods such as meat, that have been burned or browned during cooking, can cause damage to our cells' DNA (the blueprint that controls all processes[31]). Some of the chemicals from the browned portions of these foods triggered cancer when fed to rats.[32]

Cooking unsaturated fats, such as polyunsaturated margarines and cooking oils, can produce a whole chain of chemicals that promote cellular change and cancer.[33] But it isn't just the vegetable oils that can cause damage. Cholesterol, which is high in foods such as egg yolks, cheese, butter, organ meats and some fish, can also be changed by high temperature cooking into chemicals that may cause cancer.[34]

Even the brown crusty bits on the top of a loaf of bread are far from innocent. Chemicals found in bread crusts and even, I'm afraid, in toast contain DNA damaging agents that may cause cancer.[35] The browned sugar in that creme caramel is equally guilty, and coffee, which contains considerable quantities of burned coffee beans is also known to cause cellular damage[31] (heavy coffee drinking has been linked with cancers of the ovary, bladder, pancreas and colon[36]).

There is growing evidence to suggest that all the

chemicals in these over-cooked foods do their damage with a single mechanism. They lead to the formation of highly dangerous little particles called 'free radicals'. A free radical is a highly reactive particle created in the presence of oxygen (and therefore particularly common during cooking when the oxidation processes are faster). Unless controlled by the body's own anti-oxidants and anti-carcinogens, free radicals will cause not only cellular damage, cancer, and arterial hardening; they're thought to be the main cause of the ageing process too.[37]

On present evidence two cooking processes are most likely to create free radicals.[37] These are *frying*, or any process that involves heating fats and oils (especially polyunsaturated[38]), and any process that leads to *browning* or *burning*. These are the two ways of cooking to avoid. Over the years we've found ways to make food just as delicious, and three times as digestible, without having to resort to either of these dubious techniques.

Now all this doesn't mean that you take your life in your hands every time you scoff a piece of toast. Your environment and your foods (even natural uncooked ones) are full of life-threatening substances. What actually saves your life a thousand times a day is the strength of your own immune system, supplemented by the natural anti-oxidants in your diet. So far vitamin E, beta-carotene (the precursor of vitamin A), selenium, and vitamin C have been identified as natural anti-oxidants and anti-carcinogens. Building a strong immune system, and eating foods high in these nutrients (you will be doing both on the Wright Diet) should give you the protection you need to deal with any damaging chemicals you may encounter. Cutting down the assault on your immune system, however, by preparing your food with more care and respect will help you to live longer and healthier, and to look a lot younger while you're doing it.

Take Care with Equipment
The cheapest and most commonly available cookware in this country is made from aluminium. Aluminium foil is frequently used too. Now however there is growing evidence that high levels of aluminium in the brain are linked with Alzheimer's disease,[39] a very distressing form of senility which can affect people as young as 40 or 50, involving loss of memory, loss of mobility, personality changes and sometimes incontinence. Alzheimer's now kills more people in America than cancer,[40] and is becoming increasingly epidemic here too.

But aluminium cookware can also be a common cause of discomfort and bloating during digestion. This is particularly likely with acid foods such as tomatoes, rhubarb or other fruit which dissolve considerable amounts of aluminium from saucepans, and can trigger a reaction in the digestive system which leads to gas formation, bloating, stomach cramps and poor digestion. Glass and stainless steel saucepans are probably the safest. If you use tin foil make sure it doesn't come into contact with the food itself.

So far there is no evidence that microwave ovens damage the food that is cooked in them. But there is a growing suspicion that these ovens lead to a higher rate of cancer (particularly breast cancer) amongst those using them.[41] If you do use a microwave oven it's probably safer to leave the room while it's cooking. In terms of fuels I think there's very little to choose between gas and electricity. However gas is a common irritant and allergen. If you suffer from headaches or other unidentified symptoms and you have any allergic tendencies (hay fever, asthma, eczema, migraine etc.) you're probably better off with electricity.

Eat Unprocessed Foods

I once met a Canadian girl who didn't know that coffee came in any form other than 'instant' out of a jar. Today's food goes through such a sophisticated series of processes that such treatment goes almost unnoticed, or is actually thought of as normal. I frequently find myself wondering how many people really know that soups and sauces don't come out of a packet, that cream doesn't come out of an aerosol can, or that breakfast doesn't come out of a box.

But a lot of people do experience this principle for themselves. Their bodies tell them for instance that cottage cheese is easier to digest than hard cheese, because it's been through fewer processes. (By the same token a hard cheese is preferable to one that has been smoked as well!) Your own stomach will no doubt tell you that a fresh nut feels a lot more comfortable than one that has been roasted, sprayed with sugar, salt and chemicals, and kept (often for years) in a plastic or aluminium wrapping. And you should be in no doubt that a frozen pizza, probably containing synthetic cheese, and certainly the result of intense chemical processes, is going to give you a lot more trouble than a simple slice of bread and cheese.

As people begin to look for healthier ways of eating, an instinct seems to guide them to go back to the simpler foods on which the human body has always thrived. 'Real' foods are really simple. A cabbage out of the garden. A fresh fish. A loaf of homemade bread. A piece of curd cheese. An apple. A butter bean. A lamb chop.

Our Bodies Adapt Slowly

How many of us live on foods like that today? Yet this isn't nostalgic romanticism. *The truth is that these simple foods are what our bodies expect to eat.* It has taken thousands of years to evolve the ability to digest them. How can we expect to be able to handle foods transformed by dozens of chemicals and processes only invented in the last thirty years? Ten thousand years ago the more adventurous among us began to try out a new type of food.[42] One that would keep through the winter, and that could be planted and harvested (a new idea at the time), instead of having to rely on the luck of the hunters, or on the efforts of the women who went to gather roots, grubs and berries. There were several varieties of this new food – today they go by the names of wheat, oats, rice, corn, and so on – but they're all basically related to the grass family. As a group we call the edible ones 'grains'.

The fact is we're still learning how to digest these grains. Some of us, probably those descended from long lines of grain-fed ancestors, eat them without difficulty. But there are still a lot of poor grain digesters about.[43] And the result is that grains are among the most common allergens (that is they can cause allergic reactions) because many of our bodies still regard them as foreign invaders rather than as food. But if we're having trouble digesting a simple grain of wheat after ten thousand years, how can we expect to throw in half a dozen chemicals, raise it to peak temperature and pressure, spray it with oil and sugar – and then convince ourselves we've got an edible breakfast cereal?

Even flour refining is a 'process' that our bodies must adapt to, and one that involves a good deal more than the simple grinding that most of us fondly imagine. Today's white flour is matured artificially by blowing chlorine gas or other oxidising agents through it.[44] Then up to 34 other additives may be added. All this improves production, storage and profits, but is unlikely to do anything positive for our health.

The Government Can't Protect You

Don't be tempted to believe that food additives wouldn't be in use if they weren't safe. You can't expect remote government departments to take responsibility for your health; there are too many personalities and vested interests involved in decisions of that kind. Right now there are additives in use in this country that have been banned elsewhere because they're thought to cause cancer, birth defects or other health risks.[44] Most countries other than Britain don't permit the use of chlorine gas in flour for instance.

One controversial additive permitted in the UK, called BHT (used in margarines, vegetable oils, crisps, salted peanuts, breakfast cereals, and so on), is banned in many countries because it may cause reproductive failures, blood cell changes and tumour formation.[44,45] A common food colouring called Amaranth found in jams, jelly mixes and ice creams (and many other foods commonly eaten by children), as well as in some 'health' drinks and liquid vitamin C preparations, has now been banned in America, Sweden and Russia because there is sufficient evidence that it causes long-term risk to health.[46]

It has been estimated that each of us in this country now gets the equivalent of 22 aspirin-sized tablets of food additives in our diet every day. The sheer volume and complexity of the chemicals we're consuming make it impossible to know what the long-term risks may be. Had thalidomide been a slow-acting cause of cancer for instance, *it would still be in use today*. Even though the drug caused gross malformations it took almost five years of intensive research to actually prove this.

Food Additive Deception

What most of us don't realise is that the food industry can change and manipulate our food so that even our taste buds are deceived. The 'foods' *may not even contain* what we think we're tasting. Soya, maize and sugar beet, for instance, can be transformed into 'cheese', 'tomato paste' and 'salami'. They will even feel right to the mouth. Jams, yoghurts and drinks may never have seen the strawberries or the cherries that we assume from the look or the taste. And clever labelling is likely to deceive all but the quickest witted. 'Cherry flavour' for instance means what it says – that the food tastes like cherry (owing to the skilful use of chemicals), not that there are any actual cherries in it.

The manufacturers argue of course that without additives their foods would quickly spoil, and would look and taste less attractive. But that is just the point. Do we really want to eat stale food that has been made to seem fresh when it isn't? The fact that food in its natural state easily goes 'off' works for our protection. It begins to look or smell unappetising and we're naturally not tempted to eat it.

But if our taste buds are deceived, our stomachs, our bloodstream and our liver are not. Living on these foods numbs and deadens our bodies, and taxes our immunity to disease. Eventually, we begin to experience *dis-ease*.[47] Some deep-down instinct may then pull us back to the real foods. Or we may fail to pick up the signals, and continue to fossilise under the weight of preservatives, anti-oxidants, artificial colourings, and 3000 other chemical additives that the processed foods we eat may contain.

Practically speaking, to stay healthy, we need to avoid most food that comes out of tins, boxes, packets, cartons and bottles. The rule is, if it's packaged – think twice, then put it back on the shelf. Certainly never buy or use any packaged food without inspecting the label very closely. Read the list of ingredients, look up the E numbers (see Recommended Reading page 251), and unless you're really sure of the ingredients, go without. You'll probably live longer.

The Wright Diet will show you how to start clearing these chemicals and processed foods from your life. It isn't difficult. It's a question of knowing how to replace them. And this can be done very simply as you'll find when you start to follow the menus and recipes. As your body begins to clear those residues of old chemicals and accumulated poisons, you'll find you have twice the life and four times the energy.

Combine Your Foods With Care

What they don't tell you in those biology classes is that digestion isn't quite as straightforward as the textbooks suggest. The fact is that food doesn't just arrive in the stomach in neatly wrapped packages labelled 'protein', 'fat' and 'carbohydrate'. In reality, it's far more likely to arrive as a bite of hamburger, bun, chips and relish all in the same mouthful (definitely not a recipe from the Wright Diet). That's protein, fat and carbohydrate all hopelessly mixed together, which is a tall order for any stomach to tackle. Not surprisingly, there is often a compromise which results in digestion which is far from perfect.

Eating bread and cheese together for instance means that your stomach's got to tackle starch and protein in the same delivery. To begin its digestion, cheese, like all proteins, needs an *acid* environment in the stomach and the work of the enzyme pepsin (see the next chapter). But bread digestion starts in the mouth in alkaline conditions. Then it makes its way to the small intestine where it can be further broken down, again in an *alkaline* medium. Trying to do both things together is like trying to go up an escalator when everyone else is coming down. The bread grabs the action and mops up the acid (which it doesn't need) and the cheese misses out. Neither gets the treatment it really needs, and neither gets properly digested.

Starch and Protein Don't Mix Well

The clash of digestion when we stuff ourselves with meat and potatoes for instance (or with fish and rice, or omelette and chips) was first discovered sixty years ago by the American surgeon, Dr William H. Hay.[48] By withdrawing partly digested food from the stomach after meals (during which protein and starch foods had been eaten together) he was able to see what had been happening. Again and again he found that the alkaline digestion of the starch (the bread, rice, potatoes and so on) had stopped when it got to the stomach, because the level of hydrochloric acid there was high in order to digest the protein (the meat, fish, eggs, cheese etc.). Pavlov himself had already shown that the stomach secretes different levels of acid depending on how much protein is present.[49]

But when there are only starch foods in the stomach (and no proteins) the acid secreted isn't high enough to interfere with the alkaline digestive processes that have begun in the mouth. From then on the digestion of the bread, or the potatoes and so on, should have the best possible chance. Likewise, it's only when protein foods manage to get to the stomach without the competition of starches that they get enough acid to complete their first stage of digestion. From then on they should get the best chance too.

Dr Hay also showed that starch digestion can be held up when we eat what he termed the 'acid fruits' (these include apples, oranges, grapes – in fact most fruits) along with our starch foods. These fruits do however mix well with proteins. This means that eating a salad which has fruit in it when you're also having bread, rice or potatoes is likely to get you into trouble. But you can probably eat the same salad with a grilled fish or an egg without any problem. And a squeeze of lemon on that fish will positively aid its digestion by adding to the stomach's efforts to make sufficient acid. (There's a full Food Combining Chart at the back of the book.)

But what happens when you get your combinations wrong? When you throw in steak, bread and potatoes for instance, and follow it up with apple pie and cream, and then biscuits and cheese? The most immediate effect will be that your body has to work a lot harder to get the nutrients that it needs. If you've got the stomach of a Trojan this may not be much of a problem. But if you're already living at one or two degrees under, this extra stress could give you a very uncomfortable night's sleep, and probably a food combination hangover the following day. But that isn't the end of the story – you've still got to deal with the food that's left undigested or only partly digested after the battle of the combinations has done its work.

Havoc in the Bloodstream

This again is where we leave the textbooks behind. For years scientists have believed that our bodies could only absorb food once it was completely broken down into the smallest units (proteins into amino acids, carbohydrates into sugars and fats into fatty acids). But new evidence is beginning to suggest that this may not always be so – that in some conditions our bodies may in fact absorb only partly-digested food.[50] This may be one of the consequences of eating different foods together that don't digest well.

When our body absorbs a food in the undigested state, what's actually happening is that molecules that are far too long and complicated are getting into our bloodstream. Being unprepared for such a biochemical event the body reacts defensively: it treats the alien molecules as 'foreign bodies', just like invading bacteria, and quickly makes antibodies to deal with them. The next time that food is eaten and absorbed only partly digested, an 'allergic' reaction may follow.

In my experience, with my own body and my clients, you have to be already suffering discomfort, or have become particularly sensitive to your body's needs, before you really feel what good and bad food combinations are all about. (Judy Mazel, author of the Beverly Hills Diet was, from her own description, in just this condition for instance when she discovered some of the secrets of food combination for herself.) But for people suffering from problems of bloating, allergy, overweight, constant fatigue and many other symptoms which can develop from poor digestion, sorting out your food combinations can be the blessing you've been waiting for. I've known people for whom this method was the *only one*, from everything that nutritional healing has to offer, that worked for them.

Seductive Good Health

What this food combining business really comes down to is that you have to get unhooked from the idea that you must have starch and protein at every meal. We've got so fixed on this fallacy that I've known people beg for a slice of bread at a meal when there was plenty of food but no other starch being offered. Eating steak, or a grilled fish on the bone, along with a salad and nothing else, may not seem so strange. But sitting down to rice and vegetables, or to potatoes and salad, is going to seem strange to a lot of people at first. Fortunately we're creatures of habit, and habits can change. Once you've got used to the idea of having a starch *or* a protein meal, it will begin to seem the most natural and logical thing in the world.

The Wright Diet gives you the chance to see what food combining can do for you. Once you've made a start, and experienced the combinations that do work well, you're unlikely to go back to throwing it all in anyhow. The bonus, whether it's just a greater sense of ease after eating, or a radical new step forward in your life, is likely to seduce you into health whether you like it or not!

Avoid Salt And Salty Foods

As a film-struck teenager I once sat through a whole performance of *The Seven Samurai* cheerfully unaware that I'd removed my shoes the moment I sat down. When the film ended – you've probably guessed – I couldn't get them on again. There I was in the middle of Oxford Street with a pair of very puffy and unshod feet. I suspect this will be a familiar story to quite a few people. Swollen feet, swollen ankles, and even swollen fingers, are by no means uncommon (I'm not referring here to the type of swelling some women experience just before their periods). But how many people realise that this uncomfortable experience can be caused simply by eating salt?

Throughout the many millions of years of human evolution, we ate no salt. Except, that is, for the small amount found naturally in meat, fruit and vegetables. Medical estimates put the amount of salt that our bodies really need somewhere between 20 mg and 500 mg, although other researchers put this slightly higher at around 1,000 mg. Today we consume an average of somewhere between 8,000 mg and 14,000 mg every day.[51] That's somewhere between eight and twenty-eight times more than we need.

Once we'd discovered salt we soon found it was a marvellous preservative. Right up to the advent of fridges it was practically the only way you could keep meat and savoury foods fresh (sugar is the other great preserver of course.) And because salt could do this, it was highly valued for many thousands of years. In fact Roman soldiers were partly paid with it, hence the word 'salary'. It was sometimes credited with magical properties. Even today there are myths about salt. People believe for instance that they couldn't live without adding salt to their food, or that they might collapse in hot weather without it.

In fact there are tribes living healthily in jungle conditions on such low salt intakes that it's clear that neither of these beliefs can be true. It is true however that if your body is used to a lot of salt, a sudden loss through sweating in hot weather can lead to a temporary loss of equilibrium between blood and tissues that can be disturbing. But if you live on a low or salt-free diet, hot weather is no problem – you can prove that for yourself.

Most of the excess salt we eat is pushed out through the skin and the kidneys, but some is inevitably trapped in our bodies. And just like the salt left in the salt packet, this internal salt tends to collect water, and we swell. If your body's good at getting rid of salt the extra water you collect won't be very significant. But if like me you're not so good, you may take on quite a swell.

Salt is a Health Hazard

Swelling isn't the only symptom to look for however. Salt raises blood pressure, and high blood pressure can have no symptoms at all. Three out of every ten of us have high blood pressure and may not be aware of it. But high blood pressure is a risk factor for strokes and heart attacks, and six out of ten of us will die of one of those. Now, it's normal in Western countries to expect blood pressure to rise with age. But in every society (without exception) where salt is not added to the food, life-long low blood pressure is the norm. This includes the African Bushmen and Pygmies, the Brazilian Indians, the Australian Aborigines, the Eskimos and so on. And when salt is introduced into the diets of these societies then blood pressure soon starts to rise significantly.

The reason we eat so much salt (and possibly why we cling to the idea that we can't live without it) is quite simply that most of us are addicted. Salt is a stimulant. It hits the adrenal glands (see Chapter 4) and the release of adrenal hormones gives us a temporary sense of energy and well-being. But the effect doesn't last because the body readjusts. Then we want to eat something salty again. Isn't that how all addictions start?

But the knowledge that you might one day die of a

stroke is hardly likely to inhibit you, as you reach for your next packet of salted crisps. It's how you feel now that counts. If you're on a salty diet you probably can't tell how salt actually *feels* in your body. I guarantee that if you cut it out for two weeks, you will. Getting used to the lack of saltiness in your food is surprisingly easy. Your taste buds adjust very quickly. And when you do eat something salty you'll have a shock. In the first place it will taste *dreadful*. But the real surprise will come with the after-effects: that familiar old grumpy you will be back within minutes.

For me the calm and ease I feel on a low salt diet is more important than any theory. Tension is something I can do without. That doesn't mean I'm not busy and active. I am. I frequently work a fifteen-hour day, packed with meetings, brain work and deadlines. But I don't need stimulants like salt (or tea or coffee) to manage all that. Stimulants have a rebound effect. In the end they slow you down.

Use Food Supplements Wisely

The Wright Diet will almost certainly give you a higher level of essential nutrients than you were getting before you started. But there are some very good reasons why you may want to supplement your diet with extra vitamins and minerals.

Out-and-out deficiency diseases, such as scurvy or beri beri, are now rare in the Western worlds. But numerous conditions that scientists and nutritionists are beginning to recognise as 'sub-clinical' deficiencies are actually wide-spread. Frequent colds and infections, for instance, are often due to a lack of vitamin C, although they may be due to other deficiencies too, such as zinc or vitamin A. Poor skin conditions can be a sign of B vitamin deficiencies, especially when there is irritation or dry skin around the mouth, nose or eyes. Flaking nails and poor teeth may come from a diet inadequate in calcium, and so on.

The Wright Diet will put a lot of these nutrients back. But even the best quality organic foods may not give you enough to make good earlier deficiencies. In our experience, when you put your body on a healthy diet it embarks on a cleansing and healing programme that may last some time. During this period you may actually need *higher* levels of certain vitamins and minerals, because you're involved in a jump to a new level of health. Once you've attained that level (which may take a few months, or even a year or two, depending on your health before you started) your need for these nutrients will probably be reduced.

High Vitamin Primitive Diets

There are two other arguments for supplementation that I think are very important. The first is that our world is now polluted with levels of radiation and agricultural chemicals (such as DDT) as it never has been before. The human body is meeting a challenge for which it was not designed. So I take vitamins that I know will protect me, and keep my immune system strong. The other reason that persuades me to supplement my diet is the evidence left by Dr Weston Price and others about the levels of nutrients in primitive diets. Without exception the diets of the people visited by him were providing levels of vitamins and minerals *higher* than the amounts now recommended by the British or American governments.

In some cases the nutrient levels were many times higher than ours. Every one of those communities, for instance, was consuming at least 50,000 international units of vitamin A, and thriving on it.[52] Today we're told we need less than a tenth of that, and that more is dangerous! Likewise these people were regularly taking in three, four or five times as much calcium as is now recommended, and in some cases up to fifty times the level of iron.

Even the Wright Diet would find it hard to compete with such splendid nourishment. Many of these people were eating fish taken from seas that are now polluted and depleted, or eating foods that were so plain and monotonous (but high in nutrients) that only the hardiest among us would follow in their steps today. So, as an optional extra to the Wright Diet, I recommend a Basic Supplement Programme (details are given in Part Three). Don't feel that you have to use it. The remarkable benefits of the Wright Diet will be yours whether you add in the supplements or not. But the two together will definitely give you more.

In summary, the Wright Diet is based on these nine principles:

1 **Correct your acid/alkaline balance**
2 **Balance your blood sugar**
3 **Eat organically grown food when you can**
4 **Eat at least half your foods raw**
5 **Cook simply**
6 **Eat unprocessed foods**
7 **Combine your foods with care**
8 **Avoid salt and salty foods**
9 **Use food supplements wisely**

4

Getting To Know Your Body

Before you can use the Wright Diet to find the diet that's right for you, you need to get a sense of this eating business from the inside. A lot of us have the vague idea that our stomach's somewhere just south of our navel, and we manage to stuff ourselves with whatever takes our fancy year in, year out without ever wondering just what it is we're doing or why.

Certainly, knowing how the system works can help us to understand how we're made, as well as what may be going wrong. But take that knowledge and turn it into experience, *actually begin to feel what eating is about*, and we're nine tenths of the way to rediscovering that natural instinct which will always feed us perfectly, if we let it.

Anyone who has ever studied school biology has taken a trip through the digestive system at least once in their life, even if it was only what once took up the space between a French lesson and the lunch bell. In my case, because of changing schools and taking extra biology classes, I somehow managed to study the thing at least half a dozen times. I ended up thinking I knew it pretty well. But until I got in touch with the actual flesh and blood of my own body, that knowledge was just so many words and pictures inside my head.

What changed it into something that had real meaning for me was getting to know my own stomach, liver and intestines, instead of some theory out of a textbook. Then for the first time eating became a living experience. I knew what it was I was feeding, because I could feel it from the inside. And that changed the way I wanted to feed myself (that is, with more care), without any extra effort on my part.

Bringing the Body Alive

The single most shocking realisation that came to me during these 'close encounters' with my inside, was that my body is actually like a *doughnut*.

Although I knew all about the organs and structures inside me, I had been in the habit (perhaps like most of us) of using the shorthand image of my body as a sort of sack, into which I stuffed the food. But then I realised nothing could be further from the truth. I'm not a sack at all, I'm a tube! Or rather, I'm a tube with an inside and an outside, just like a doughnut. My inner tube is my digestive system which travels from my mouth to my anus. And the skin of my body is the outside of the doughnut.

So when food goes down into my stomach *it still isn't inside me*. It's just parked in the middle of the doughnut. And that whole territory on the inside of the digestive tube is really a kind of no-man's land where battle is done between armies of enzymes, bacteria, digestive juices and the food I eat (see the diagram on page 90). Only at the end of the battle is the loot, the digested food, sneaked into my body through the walls of the small intestine. Getting to know myself as this tall doughnut has really helped bring my body (and my experience of feeding it) alive.

Most of us give very little time to developing an awareness of the inside of our bodies. Perhaps because we're all so busy with the world around us, or perhaps because we've been taught to believe that focusing on ourselves is self-indulgent. But there's nothing more self-indulgent than getting ill, or failing to reach our full potential, because we don't have the instinct to take care of ourselves properly.

There are actually very few experiences that enhance the quality of life quite as much as being fully in touch with the warm human body in which we're living.

Tuning In

Developing this awareness often involves starting by tuning in to the parts that hurt. The first part of my body that forced itself on my attention was the area under my right ribcage. That area turned out to be my liver and another very troublesome little organ called the gall bladder that is tucked into a fold of it. Both of them, I discovered, were getting upset and angry at the way I was treating them. When I fed them cucumbers they would wince and turn critical; wine made them hot and argumentative; and when I ate cheese they became soggy and depressed. With my new awareness of these tetchy organs, and using the Wright Diet, I have changed what I eat to make them (and me) feel a thousand times better.

The second area to make its presence known was the middle of my back. Sometimes I'd feel a collapsed sensation there that would make it hard to sit at a table without slumping on my elbows. At other times I would feel anxiety and tension in just the same area. The organs responsible for this fuss were actually my kidneys, and two hypersensitive little glands perched right on top of them, called my adrenal glands. My kidneys and adrenal glands, I finally discovered, hate salt. Salt makes them snarl and spit. Then my back aches and my hands and feet swell. If I eat enough of it my body takes on water as if it's expecting a siege.

This was a tough one for me because I've been a salt

freak all my life. You could forget the biscuits and the ice cream. Give me a packet of salted crisps any time! But once I had inner contact with those organs in my back I couldn't devour the crisps or the salt in quite the same way. As soon as I did I heard the 'Ouch!' So cutting out salt was quite easy after all. Now I have a back that's relaxed and strong, with the occasional grunt when a little salt slips past my watchdog. I weigh a lot less too, without all that extra swell on board.

Contacting my other organs wasn't quite so easy. None of them were quite as vociferous as my liver and friends. I had to wait for the cross ones to quieten down before I could get a real sense of the others. Sometimes I would actually talk to them: 'Hello there, stomach, can you hear me?' And sometimes I'd get a reply: 'Hmmm! Yes, what do you want?' or 'Aaah, I'm very comfortable, thank you!' Now I know them all. My stomach, my pancreas, my liver, my gall bladder, my small intestine, my colon, my kidneys, my heart, my lungs and so on. I can feel them, I hear their needs, and I'm letting them teach me how to feed and take care of myself.

How to Start
Start getting to know your body better by studying the diagram on page 90.

Don't worry about what all the different parts do. Come back to details like that when you want to know more. Remember you're not trying to store yet more facts in your head. The object of the exercise is to become more aware of the signals – be they aches and pains or sensations of relaxation and pleasure – that you're already getting from your body, and in particular from your digestive system and major organs. Getting clearer and stronger signals from your body by doing this is the most important step you can take towards letting your body tell you what it needs and what it doesn't.

Start with the digestive system. When you have a basic idea of how the digestive system is built, find a quiet place and ten minutes when you won't be disturbed. (The only essential is that you should be able to concentrate without distraction – you can sit and do it on a bus or in a traffic jam so long as you give it your sole attention.) Close your eyes and go inside.

Try to feel your way down the digestive system inside you, starting with your mouth, your throat, the tube down to your stomach and so on. Don't worry if you can't actually feel your stomach or some other organ straight away. That will come in time. Open your eyes and check with the diagram whenever you need to.

After a while of course you won't need to work from the diagram because you'll be aware of the real thing inside you. And once you feel you're in touch with your digestive system, start bringing in the other organs by working with the diagram on page 95 too.

Feeling Your Digestion

Most people have scant knowledge of their digestive process. 'It's fine,' they tell me, 'really no problem.' Then they add casually that they do suffer some discomfort after eating, or that they sometimes get a little bloated and distended. Or they remember to tell me that they frequently suffer from wind, or perhaps that they've been constipated for most of their life, or even that they get diarrhoea every morning. What astonishes me is that many of these confidences are given to me as after-thoughts – that so many people can have such experiences and still believe that their digestion is 'fine'.

This happens of course because most of us are out of

touch with what's going on when we digest our food. We don't associate one piece of our experience – actually eating – with what happens some time later, such as becoming bloated or constipated. So we don't see that one follows the other. And that discomfort or distension is trying to tell us something about our food or the way we're digesting it.

Digesting a meal from beginning to end takes a minimum of twelve hours. That is from seeing it on the plate, to eliminating what the body doesn't want. A twelve-hour transit time however is exceptional for anyone eating conventional Western food. Lack of fibre and high levels of gluten (a very sticky protein found in wheat) can slow the transit time down to one, two or three days, sometimes even longer. Throughout that time it's possible to remain conscious of your body, and of what effect the food is having on you as a whole. I don't mean of course that you should think about nothing else. On the contrary, you don't want to get obsessive. Just tune in on a regular basis and pick up the signals as to what's going on.

Inevitably you'll start noticing the uncomfortable times. Moments of cramp or distension perhaps, slight sensations of nausea, dull aches and pains, the experience of swelling or bloating, or the sense of shut-down that comes with constipation. To begin with just allow yourself to become more aware of these experiences – that awareness in itself will begin a healing process.

Once you feel more in touch with the feeling of your digestion, take another look at the digestion diagrams and start to identify the organs that are most sensitive. Is your discomfort in the area of your stomach for instance, or much lower down – in your small intestine perhaps, or even in your colon? The times of transit given on the diagram will give you extra clues too. If your first moment of discomfort comes within two or three hours after eating, the problem is probably located in your duodenum. If it's sooner than that you may have a fussy stomach. If you wake up in the night with pain many hours after eating, or the pain is always low in your abdomen then you might have trouble with your small intestine or colon.

It may seem a pointless exercise to become more aware of where you hurt. Most people take frequent painkillers to achieve just the opposite. But surprising as it may seem, becoming more aware of your aches and pains is the only way you can ever hope to be finally free of them. That instinct was lost in childhood as we each *cut off* from the experience of our body. Getting back into your body again will reawaken that instinct so that you are once more in touch with your needs, feelings and internal experience.

The Right Diet for Your Body

There is a good reason for all of this. Becoming more aware of your body will help to improve your health. From the moment you begin the Wright Diet you'll start to feel changes. Internally you'll feel cleaner, clearer and more alive. And as you do, you'll become more aware of the parts of you that still don't feel so good. This is where the awareness exercises are important. They'll help you to focus more precisely on what is giving you trouble, so that you can begin to heal yourself.

And you do that by changing your diet until your body responds – until your aches and pains vanish, until your energy rises, until your digestion feels good all the way through, and until your body as a whole feels comfortable, alive and full of optimism.

For this you need the Food Tests on page 112. When

you do the Food Tests you eliminate different foods from your diet in a sequence that allows you to discover which foods give you discomfort and which don't. Absurd as it may seem, this simple exercise holds a major key to your health and wholeness. Whatever aches, pains, skin problems, digestive difficulties, or emotional troubles (such as anxiety or depression) you may have, the chances are that your diet has something to do with it.

Many symptoms, however unlikely, can be caused directly by food intolerance – from chronic earache, bed wetting and sinus conditions to eczema, some forms of arthritis, and schizophrenia[53]. The list is endless. But even if your condition is not caused specifically by a food problem, there are ways you can change your diet to help it. This is the basis of nutritional healing. And this is why the Wright Diet will help you, whatever your need.

The Value of Fasting

Once a week during the Wright Diet you take a day of rest and renewal on a very simple diet – your Fast Day. It isn't obligatory but I do recommend it. A fast will not only help to tune you to your internal experience. It will heal, cleanse and recharge you too.

The Wright Diet is a cleansing experience in itself of course. Your body will begin to throw off toxins and accumulated sludge from the moment you start. But when you discover what fasting on vegetables, fruit and juices can do for you, I think you will be overjoyed. For this is the final secret that nutrition has to offer – that fasting is one of the ultimate healers.

This 'secret' has actually been known for thousands of years. Every ancient tradition knew that fasting healed many disorders, beautified the skin, reduced your waistline and kept you young. But of course we have forgotten it. Now we have to learn again what our great grandmothers probably knew as a simple truth.

Today we have become so convinced that we must eat three meals a day to stay healthy, that it's hard for us to believe that not doing so for a short time can actually make you healthier. On the Wright Diet you need have no anxiety. You don't have to stop eating, just change what you eat. Nor should you ever feel hungry. Fast Days on the Wright Diet are carefully balanced so that your body can cleanse and eliminate, while you feel good at the same time.

Cleansing and Healing

Unless we live on a very pure and alkaline diet our bodies tend to accumulate toxins. These can be chemicals such as certain food additives and pesticides, heavy metals such as lead, or old drug residues (both medical and self-administered). Our body processes also produce waste materials, and when elimination is sluggish, these can build up in our tissues.

Toxins are not particularly pleasant to live with. They can cloud your brain, make you heavy and sluggish, and give you dull and spotty skin. But when you get rid of them you'll feel as alive and as vital as you did when you were a child. You'll also shed excess weight and water; your skin will heal and soften; and your brain will clear – you'll discover that you can actually think and make decisions again.

Fasting can do this for you because it dramatically speeds the elimination of toxins. When you eat only simple alkaline foods, you reach a point at which the body switches to another mode – it begins to fast. During fasting the remains of old body cells are swiftly broken down and replaced. Organs and systems in need of healing are given prompt attention. Toxins and excess fluid are eliminated. Skin cells are replaced. At every level of the body, the rate of healing is rapidly accelerated.

It's quite normal to get a mild headache or the occasional twinge of nausea when fasting. These are signs that the fast is working and that your liver and tissues are throwing off toxins and having a good springclean. Drink plenty of spring or filtered water (to which you might add a dash of fresh lemon – it helps the cleansing) and the sensations will soon pass. Occasionally more severe cleansing reactions are experienced. In such a case, give yourself the time to rest, break your fast very gently with simple foods and choose a less rigorous fasting menu the next time.

Because the interior and the exterior of our lives always reflect each other your Fast Day might best coincide with the day you spend cleaning your home, seeing to your laundry, sorting out your finances or having a good bonfire in the garden. It can of course be a day of work instead, but whatever kind of day you spend you will find that the effect of the fast will be to draw you inwards to an increased inner awareness and understanding. When you break your fast the next day you should feel renewed and ready for the world once more.

Your Digestive System

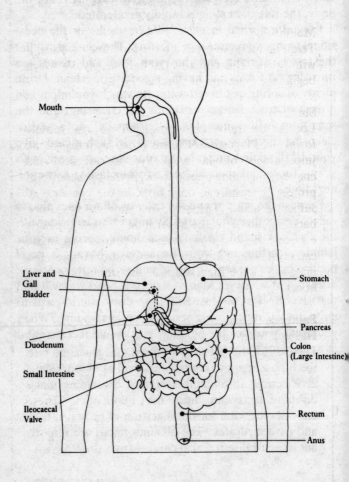

Mouth

Liver and
Gall
Bladder

Stomach

Duodenum

Pancreas

Colon
(Large Intestine)

Small Intestine

Ileocaecal
Valve

Rectum

Anus

Key to Your Digestive System

Mouth
Teeth and tongue break up the food and combine it with saliva. This contains the enzyme ptyalin which begins the digestion of starches.

Stomach
Located centrally just below your ribcage. Mainly for protein digestion. Churns food. Secretes gastric juice which contains weak hydrochloric acid and enzymes including pepsin to begin the breakdown of protein. (Pepsin can only work in the presence of sufficient acid.) The acid also protects by killing bacteria and helps the absorption of some minerals e.g. calcium and iron. Water, alcohol and glucose can be absorbed directly into bloodstream here. The majority of the meal stays in the stomach for 3–5 hours.

Pancreas
Has two functions:
1. Releases the hormones insulin and glucagon into the bloodstream to control the level of blood sugar.
2. Releases an alkaline secretion containing many digestive enzymes into the duodenum. These enzymes are vital for the digestion of proteins, fats, and carbohydrates. The alkaline juices are important to neutralise the acid coming from the stomach.

continued overleaf

Key to Your Digestive System – *cont.*

Liver and Gall Bladder

The liver makes bile – an alkaline juice containing bile pigments (which come from broken-down red blood cells and give the colour to our faeces). Bile is stored in the gall bladder and released into the duodenum when fat is being eaten, to help its digestion. The liver turns digested food into substances our body will need, and stores them. Body chemicals are broken down here and their ingredients recycled. Drugs and poisons can be detoxified and excreted in the bile.

Duodenum and Small Intestine

Food mixes with the bile and alkaline juices and enzymes from the pancreas as they pour into the duodenum (the first 10 inches of the small intestine). Digested food begins to be absorbed into the bloodstream and lymph vessels (food actually begins to enter the body here). The small intestine secretes more digestive enzymes completing protein, sugar, starch and fat digestion. The whole surface of the small intestine is designed like a giant towel to soak up and absorb as much digested food as possible. Total length about 21 feet. Food takes approximately 4–7 hours to pass through the small intestine.

Key to Your Digestive System – *cont.*

Colon or Large Intestine
The colon's function is to absorb water and minerals from the residues left in the system (now becoming the faeces). It supports a colony of helpful bacteria known as the 'flora' which help make some B vitamins and vitamin K, and which make up at least a third of the bulk. They also keep the intestines 'sweet', preventing putrefaction and bad-smelling wind. Some of the bacteria that make up the flora have been shown to have natural antibiotic and anti-cancer properties. About 5 feet long. Food residues may begin to reach the anus twelve hours after eating, but total transit time may be as long as two or three days if there is constipation.

Ileocaecal Valve
This valve at the junction between the small intestine and the colon prevents the contents of the colon from getting back to the intestines.

Rectum and Anus
This normally remains empty. The feeling of distension brings about defecation. The anus consists of bands of voluntary and involuntary muscles which must relax to allow faeces to exit.

continued overleaf

Key to Your Digestive System – *cont.*

Enzymes
Enzymes are natural chemicals that help to speed body processes. The mouth, the stomach, the pancreas and the small intestine all secrete enzymes which help to break down (or in other words digest) proteins, fats or carbohydrates.

Structure
The whole digestive tract is lined with a mucus membrane which secretes mucus to lubricate the food and protect the lining itself from being digested (which would cause an ulcer). The entire tube is supported by layers of muscle which contract in waves to move the food. Nerves are supplied to the whole system to control the muscle movements and the digestive processes.

Your Other Organs

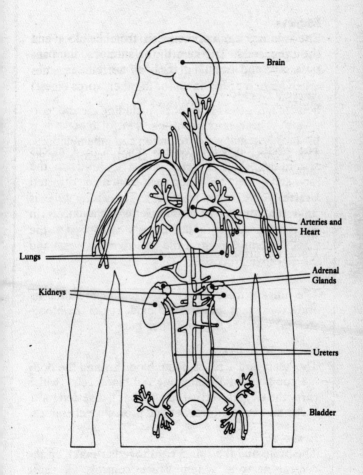

Brain

Arteries and Heart

Lungs

Adrenal Glands

Kidneys

Ureters

Bladder

Key to Your Other Organs

Kidneys
The kidneys clear waste material from the blood into the urine, and help to keep the balance of sodium and potassium and the fluid of the body constant.

Adrenal Glands
Secrete anti-stress hormones, including natural 'cortisone'. These hormones help control blood sugar balance, salt and water retention and inflammations. The kidneys and the adrenal glands have a strong influence on blood pressure.

Ureters
Take the urine to the bladder for elimination.

Bladder
Holds the urine until elimination.

Lungs
The lungs extract oxygen from the air breathed in, and exchange it for carbon dioxide (from the bloodstream) which is then breathed out.

Heart and Arteries
The heart and arteries pump blood around the body – a complex fluid containing red blood cells (which carry the oxygen and carbon dioxide), digested food, waste materials, hormones and protective chemicals.

Brain
The brain and the spinal cord together make up the central nervous system which controls all sense perceptions and muscle movements of the body.

Your Bowel Movements

Healthy faeces leave the body in an easy-flowing movement all of one piece. They break up as they leave the body, and should actually start to disintegrate once in the water, but they shouldn't consist of several compacted pieces grafted together, as is common. Compacted faeces indicate a lack of fibre in your diet and/or poor bacterial function.

Faeces should float. If they don't you're producing too much mucus – a sure sign of irritation, probably due to food intolerance (so watch for changes when you do the Food Tests).

The ideal colour is lightish brown. If they're yellow or chalky in colour you're not producing enough bile from the gall bladder (this may well change during the Food Tests). If they're very dark the food you're eating isn't right for you either.

There's no need for faeces to be foul smelling. Again this means you're on the wrong foods. Faeces do have a natural smell however. Once you've identified the odour of your own healthy faeces you'll get a daily feedback of how well you're feeding yourself.

There's no rule about how often you should have a bowel movement, so don't get obsessive about it. When you're at your best, however, you can expect one two or three times a day. This will only happen

continued overleaf

Your Bowel Movements – *cont.*

when you're getting a good amount of fibre in your diet, and when your colon bacterial population is thriving.

It's possible to 'tag' your food so you can tell how long it's taking to get through the body. A sprinkling of whole sesame seeds on a meal, or a glass of beetroot juice are two good ways of doing this. Then look for the sesame seeds or a beetroot colour to come through in the faeces.

5
The Wright Diet
Stage One: The Diet

Within days of starting the Wright Diet your skin will be glowing, your head will be clearing and your body will be feeling a new kind of strength. Your health problems too will be on the retreat, your excess weight will be slipping away and you'll be starting to feel a new and younger you.

This diet will take you further than any existing health diet so far. The only diet that can take you farther is the final stage of the Wright Diet itself – the Food Tests from which you will develop your own perfect diet. When you're ready for that step, your prospects for health and well-being will be truly unlimited. But first you must start at the beginning, with the first stage of the Wright Diet – your bridge from the old way of eating to the new.

Restocking Your Kitchen
You'll probably want to start by completely restocking your kitchen. I remember one glorious day when I went through every single item of food in our kitchen and threw out everything that wasn't actually 'real'. Out went the sticky old sauce bottles, the packets of custard powder, the tins of spaghetti, the packet puddings and a whole lot more. When I'd finished there was just a small pile of vegetables and fruit, some whole grain flour and rice, a bag of dried apricots, a jar of honey, some cheeses and two herring. That experience alone felt like a watershed. What had we been eating all those years? Clearly not 'food' in the true sense at all.

But going without some of your favourite foods – just like that – can be really tough. If you're anything like me you treat food as comfort and feel quite threatened when someone tries to take it away. That's exactly what can happen at this point of transition. Yet until you give yourself the chance to go without all those chemical, denatured and addictive foods you'll never find out just how good your body can feel without them. And then you'll never reach the stage at which your body just doesn't want to eat that way any more.

The Feast Day

So the Wright Diet has a built-in Feast Day, once every seven days. On your Feast Day you can eat anything you like, and especially those foods you've been craving all through the week. This isn't just indulgence. It serves a real purpose. You've only got to try it to understand. One woman wrote to me for instance, 'I was shocked at how differently I felt about chocolate and ice cream after my first Feast Day. I don't know if I can face either of them again for quite a while!'

Then there will be all the new foods for you to experience – succulent fresh raw vegetable salads, sprouted whole green lentils, energy-packed seeds such as pumpkin and sunflower, and delicious new grains like buckwheat and barley. Even now, I'm still discovering more. There are exciting new ways to cook and prepare it all too – easy raw food dishes, oh-so digestible ways of oil-free cooking, vegetables steamed to tasty perfection, inspiring fish dishes, mouth-watering desserts. Nouvelle cuisine – eat your heart out!

Experiment with Foods

It's very important, at this stage, to explore the widest range of foods that you can. But don't force yourself –

don't eat anything you don't like. You're trying to develop an instinct, not suppress it – and 'not liking' is usually very good instinct at work. But if you're going to evolve the right diet for you, your body has to taste the foods it's going to choose from. Until you're really sure you don't like a food, give it a fair trial.

You can stay on stage one of the Wright Diet for as long as feels comfortable. Two weeks or two years. But when you feel ready – perhaps when you sense that Stage One has taken you as far as it can – then you're ready for Stage Two of the Wright Diet – the Food Tests (see the next chapter). Using the Food Tests you'll make your way to your own Wright Diet.

The Wright Diet: Week One

The first week of the Wright Diet is a week of cleansing and reorientation. Days One and Two are simply two days of very healthy eating. They start you on the cleansing process and allow you to adjust gently to Days Three, Four and Five, which are days when you fast on a delicious variety of fresh fruit and vegetables. You break your fast on Day Six with two more days of good simple eating before you're ready to start Week Two.

Week One is a time for enjoyment and discovery. You'll begin to experience for yourself the first hint of what can be achieved. You'll lose weight of course, but more important still, you'll start to lose toxins. By Day Seven you'll probably be looking and feeling a good deal better than you have in years. Your skin, your hair and your eyes will be glowing, your head will be clear as a bell, and you should be feeling marvellous.

This week is also one of withdrawal. You won't be

drinking tea or coffee (you can go back to them in Week Two), and you'll be eating very little wheat or dairy products. Removing all these for just one week gives your body a chance to adjust and establish itself before you begin the work of finding the diet that really suits you.

In the first two or three days you may experience a headache as your body purges and eliminates all that unwanted waste. You may also feel quite tired, especially if you have been a heavy coffee drinker. Both reactions are absolutely fine. Drink lots of good fresh water and take yourself off to bed at an outrageously early hour. Let yourself go right down into the tiredness. You'll come up smiling and five years younger at the other end.

Twice during the week take a long hot bath with four ounces of bicarbonate of soda to help the cleansing process. Get a loofah and rub yourself briskly all over, as hard as feels good, especially over areas of cellulite. A sauna would be good too if you have access to one. Try to take a good brisk walk every day too, of at least half an hour.

If you have decided to take the Basic Supplement Programme, start it now, each morning with your breakfast (see page 231 for details).

DAY ONE

To Start the Day

A glass of hot water with a squeeze of fresh lemon,
or springwater and fresh lemon
or just hot or cold water.

Note: Use only filtered water or springwater for drinks and cooking, especially during Week One and when fasting. Don't drop slices of lemon complete with peel into your drinks unless they're unsprayed.

Breakfast

A selection of fresh fruit, or just one kind if you prefer. Slice open a melon for instance and scoop spoonfuls straight from the fruit, or treat yourself to a pineapple, or chop a fruit salad and dress it with a little springwater and lemon juice *or* any fresh raw vegetables. Choose from crunchy carrots, stalks of celery, slices of green pepper, whole baby tomatoes etc.

If you can get them, sprinkle two dessertspoons of ground linseeds on to your fruit or fruit salad, or stir them into fruit juice and drink them down. The linseeds are excellent for helping digestion, and marvellous for your skin, but they also help to prevent constipation – essential while you're cleansing!

Take your Basic Supplement Programme (optional).

Mid-morning Snack

Throughout the morning you can snack on any of the items listed under breakfast. You can also nibble on sunflower and pumpkin seeds.

Drink any fruit or vegetable juices, preferably freshly pressed, but if you don't have a juicer make sure you buy ones that are free of sugar, salt and preservatives. (If they come in an aluminium carton decant them into something else as soon as you open them.) You can also drink springwater and hot or cold filtered water (with lemon if you prefer). You won't be drinking any tea or coffee this week but you can add one teaspoon of honey to hot water and lemon if you wish.

Lunch
Select a large raw vegetable salad or vegetable crudités
with dressing from the recipe section, and serve it with
humous
or potato salad or baked potato
or a bean salad
or tabbouli salad
(see the recipe section for all of these)

Mid-afternoon Snack
As mid-morning. You can go on nibbling all afternoon if
you like. Remember to keep drinking water and juices.

Dinner
A large raw vegetable salad (choose from any in the
recipe section) with dressing, served with
baked or grilled fish (not smoked)
or a simple serving of goat's or cottage cheese
or a bean casserole
or 2 oz of any nuts and seeds
or any of the dishes listed under lunch

Evening Snacks
Fruit, raw vegetables, seeds, water and juices only.

DAY TWO

As Day One

DAY THREE

Fast Day.
Select your meals from the Fast Day Menu Plan given
opposite.

Fast Day Menu Plan

To Start the Day

A glass of hot water with a squeeze of fresh lemon, *or* springwater and lemon *or* just hot or cold water.

Note: Use only filtered water or springwater for drinks and cooking, while fasting. Don't drop lemon slices complete with peel into your drinks unless they're unsprayed.

Breakfast

A selection of fresh fruit, or just one kind if you prefer. Feast on half a pound of grapes, gorge yourself on a mango, munch on an apple or help yourself to any other fruit that takes your fancy. Or take the time to chop a delicious fruit salad dressed with springwater and lemon.

Or any fresh raw vegetables. Choose from crunchy carrots, stalks of celery, slices of green pepper, whole baby tomatoes etc. as during Week One. Take your linseeds with breakfast if you are able to get them, and continue your Basic Supplement Programme.

Snack on fruit or vegetables freely throughout the morning. Drink plenty of springwater, fruit juices, and hot or cold water and lemon.

continued overleaf

Fast Day Menu Plan – *cont.*

Lunch
Select a raw vegetable salad from the recipes but dress it only with a little lemon juice or not at all if you prefer.

Or a vegetable soup made without added oil (see the recipes).

Or continue to eat fresh fruit and vegetables as you have throughout the morning. You can snack on these throughout the afternoon. Remember to drink plenty of springwater, hot or cold filtered water and juices.

Dinner
Make another large raw vegetable salad and serve it with a baked potato
or brown rice and steamed vegetables
or buckwheat and steamed vegetables
or a portion of humous
(see the recipes.)
Use no dressing other than a squeeze of lemon on the salad or the potato.

Or you can continue to fruit fast into the evening or just snack on fresh vegetables if you prefer.

Remember to drink plenty of springwater, hot or cold filtered water and juices.

DAY FOUR

As Day Three

DAY FIVE

As Day Three

DAY SIX

As Day One

DAY SEVEN

As Day One

NOTE   If you felt good about the healing and cleansing that you gained from Week One of the Wright Diet you can repeat it, but don't do it for at least six weeks after the first time.

Week Two

DAYS ONE TO SIX

Select all meals from the Wright Diet Menu Plan.

The Wright Diet Menu Plan

For full details of which foods are permitted in the Wright Diet, and which are restricted please turn to page 173.

Breakfast
Select any breakfast from the recipe section.
Sprinkle two dessertspoons of ground linseeds on to whichever breakfast you choose.
Take your Basic Supplement Programme (optional).

Mid-Morning Snacks
Choose any of the fruit, nut or seed snacks given in the recipe section.

Lunch
Select any of the meals from the recipe section.

Mid-Afternoon Snack
Choose any of the snacks (including grain snacks) from the recipe section.

Dinner
Select any of the meals from the recipe section.

Evening Snacks
Choose any of the fruit, nut or seed snacks from the recipe section.

continued overleaf

The Wright Diet Menu Plan – *cont.*

Drinks

Springwater, filtered water, fruit and vegetable juices.

Grain coffees, herb teas.

Tea and coffee within your daily allowance:

coffee (ground), 1 daily; tea, 2 daily; decaffeinated coffee, 3 daily.

Alcohol: daily maximum 1 glass of wine, or ½ pint of real beer of ½ pint organic cider (Aspall's). No spirits.

No chocolate drinks, instant coffee or cola drinks.

DAY SEVEN

Your first Feast Day! You can eat and drink whatever you like. See below.

Your Feast Day

Once a week on the Wright Diet plan a Feast Day. This is a day when you break all the rules and take any food or drink that you like. Believe it or not, this is not an indulgence but a carefully designed strategy that will actually help your transition to a healthier diet.

The Feast Day is a day to treat yourself to whatever you fancy, and especially to anything you have been craving. A large helping of Black Forest gâteau perhaps or a delicious piece of Camembert cheese. Of course there is absolutely no need to force yourself to eat any of these things if you have no desire for them. Your Feast Day may be a much more simple affair: an ice cream perhaps and a cup of hot chocolate.

As you continue your Feast Days you will find that they change. Your desires will become simpler and more balanced as your body stabilises. You'll discover that you don't really enjoy a lot of the food that you once craved.

Week Three

Week Three and all following weeks have a similar but flexible structure. You can arrange each week to suit your lifestyle. For five of the seven days select your meals and snacks from the recipe section. Your Wright Diet days can be *any* of the seven days. They don't have to be the first five. For instance, they could be Days One, Two and Three and then Days Five and Seven. Or any other arrangement that suits you.

The other two days of the week are a Fast Day and a Feast Day. Both are optional but strongly recommended.

Your Fast Day is a day of cleansing and renewal. Many people find that Sunday is a good day for this, but you can choose any day that you like. It doesn't have to be the same day every week, although you may find yourself slipping into a pattern that works well.

On your Feast Day you can eat whatever you like. Time it to coincide with a day when you're spending time with friends, or going to a party, or perhaps save it for when you can be all alone and really indulge yourself. Don't have a Feast Day straight after a Fast Day, but the other way around is fine.

Once you have spent three weeks on the Wright Diet you can begin the Food Tests given in Chapter 6 (or you can carry on with the regular Wright Diet for as long as you wish). When doing Food Tests follow the sequence of days given for them and come back to the regular Wright Diet when you finish.

6

The Wright Diet
Stage Two: The Food Tests

The Wright Diet will transform your health, recharge your batteries and make you feel yourself again. It may also clear a skin problem, improve your digestion, help you shed weight, and so on; the result for each person will be different, depending on how closely the Wright Diet matches your ideal. Over the last few years, however, I have been developing a method which allows you to go beyond the Wright Diet, or any other 'health' diet, to discover the diet that is right for you in every detail. This diet – your own Wright diet – can give you unlimited health. To reach it you must take the Wright Diet Food Tests.

Essentially the Tests are an extension of the way I have always worked intuitively with my own body. Over a period of time I find I become more conscious of my body's needs and imbalances, then I look to see how the foods I'm eating are helping to increase or decrease those factors. Although I would never claim that food and drink are the only cause of aches, pains and other symptoms – whether physical, emotional, or mental – I have found that food plays a surprising part, and that this aspect of healing is generally most neglected.

Your Body will Tell You
I remember a time when I used to get a headache practically every afternoon. It was a feeling of tightness around the forehead that made thinking like trying to run

through cotton wool. I'd probably been living with the headache for a long time before it floated up and presented itself. From then on I could see just how disabling it was. Basically I wasn't getting anything done in the afternoons. When people tried to talk to me all they were getting were woolly answers.

Around the same time I was cutting down on my coffee drinking because it seemed to be making me jumpy. In fact I was down to just one cup a day. The real thing, of course, from freshly ground beans, at around eleven o'clock each morning. I don't know what made me put two and two together. But this is where intuition can be very useful. I just remember standing there one day, inhaling the fabulous smell of the beans I was grinding and being almost certain that this next cup of coffee was going to give me that headache.

It did. I proved it by stopping my coffee for several days and then trying it again. I found I could stop and start my headaches just like that. I had the same experience with several other foods over the years, and removed them from my diet or reduced them considerably, to the vast improvement of my health. The Wright Diet Tests will do the same for you – help connect your food and your reactions in a similar way. The only difference is that you won't have to stumble over clues as I did in the early days. Nor will you have to rely on intuition. The Tests do all that for you. All you need do is to notice what you're eating, and stay aware of how you and your body feel.

Understand Your Needs Better
This stage of the diet also gives you the opportunity to find out which way of nourishment really suits you best. Your ideas about what's right or healthy for you could be completely turned around. You may find that you flourish

on a grain-based diet for instance, or you may categorically decide that it's not for you. You may learn that your vegetarian ideals don't suit your stomach, and that you thrive on protein from meat and fish. Or you may discover that you feel wonderful on nothing but vegetables.

You may even come to the conclusion that fruit doesn't suit you. Last year a client came to see me because she suffered from terrible bloating and distension. Whenever she felt really bad she would fast on fruit with the idea that this was right for her, although it rarely made her better. I suggested that fruit might be the very last thing for her particular needs and worked out a very low carbohydrate diet until she felt better. She phoned a month later to say she was completely cured and was now only eating fruit with caution.

But you shouldn't miss the chance to test your reaction to individual foods as well. You may discover for instance that tomatoes have been triggering the indigestion or the joint pain you've been suffering for years. Some of your foods may be causing weight gain or bloating. Others may assault you with a woolly head or a bout of depression.

Just how much of this detective work you want to do right now will depend on your needs. Your newly developed awareness of your internal body messages may be throwing up quite a few symptoms you'd like to be rid of. Or you may be feeling that stage one of the Wright Diet is quite enough change for the time being. That's fine. We each of us have our own pace. The Food Tests are ready when you are. Just keep working on your awareness and don't force yourself to do anything.

Unmasking Reactions to Foods

Over two thousand years ago Hippocrates, the Greek, noticed that if you stop eating a food for four days or longer, you may get a reaction when you eat that food again. Doctors working on allergy and food intolerance have rediscovered the same principle: stopping a food for several days exaggerates a reaction that might otherwise go undetected. And just because a reaction is undetected, or 'masked', doesn't mean that your health isn't being affected. For instance, if you came out in a rash when you were first given eggs as a child, the chances are that you're still sensitive. But by now your reaction will be masked. Rediscovering your reaction to eggs by taking Food Test 3 could help you solve a skin problem, get rid of your headaches, or help you lose weight. You won't know what the results might be until you try.

It doesn't matter what these reactions are caused by. Some will be allergies, some will be digestive failures, some will be inabilities to deal with difficult chemicals. All you have to do is to become aware of them, and then learn which foods are responsible.

What Reactions are You Looking For?

Before you start the tests you need a most important piece of equipment. A notebook. Begin by making a list of all the aspects of your physical, emotional and mental health that you would like to improve. At the top of the list might be weight loss or freedom from depression for instance. Include even small items that bother you such as a patch of athlete's foot or a little flatulence. There is no guarantee that all of these symptoms will turn out to be nutritional problems. But they may be, and the process of writing your list will sharpen your internal perceptions.

Once you begin a Food Test you must start a food diary in your notebook (overleaf). At the end of the withdrawal phase in particular, when you start to eat those foods again, you must write down everything that you eat and drink, and record the time and how you are feeling throughout the day. The symptoms to record are the ones you're interested in changing. The food diary may seem like a neurotic nightmare or it may fascinate you. Either way you will learn a great deal. This is how you do it:

Food Diary

1 Put the date in column 1
2 Put the time of each diary entry in column 2
3 Put all foods and drinks in column 3
4 Put any reactions in column 4

DATE	TIME	FOOD & DRINKS	SYMPTOMS
18/9/85	8.30	Porridge and honey	Fine
	9.15	Tea without milk	slight headache
	10.30	Banana bread	Feeling good
	12.30	Humous and Green Farm Salad	Tight headache for 2–3 hours (humous?) Perhaps I'm sensitive to chickpeas –

The Withdrawal Phase

While you're cutting out the foods in a Test you may get certain reactions. The most common is a headache. This is an excellent sign. Your headache means you're experiencing withdrawal symptoms from one or more of the foods that you're excluding. And that means your test will probably bear fruit, and provide you with clues that could free your health and your energy from something that's been affecting you. Stay with the headache if you can and don't take painkillers. Drink lots of springwater, with a little fresh lemon if you prefer, and wait for it to pass before beginning retesting.

Retesting Phase

Once you start retesting foods you may well get quite a spectrum of reactions. In the first place it's important that you identify them and make a note in your Food Diary. But you don't want to suffer more than you need. Again drinking plenty of good water helps. But you can also shorten a reaction by taking five or ten grams of vitamin C (not sustained release in this case), and digestive enzyme supplements (from good health shops) which will also help a great deal. Take two to four immediately, and repeat both the enzymes and the vitamin C every two hours.

It's important that you don't try any more of the Test foods until the reaction to the last one has passed.

Taking Action

As soon as you start discovering the foods that affect you, you're probably going to start feeling guilty if you don't give them up right away. Don't. There's absolutely no need to force yourself to do anything, and there's certainly no need to feel guilty. You have an inbuilt instinct to help you stop taking foods and other things that hurt you. All you have to do is to let yourself be part of that natural process. When you do it this way you'll find it isn't difficult at all.

For instance grapes, raisins, wine and the other foods in Test 9 give me dreadful head and liver aches. So I avoid them like the plague. Practically every week someone tries to commiserate with me because I'm missing such treats. But that's not the case at all. These foods aren't treats for me. They hurt. Once my body fully experienced this, it was a pleasure to stop eating and drinking them, and go pain-free for the first time in my life. I didn't do it overnight of course. I went off and on the foods quite a few times until I was really sure I didn't enjoy them. You can do the same. Keep eating that food until it's *the food itself that gives you up*.

It may not come to that of course. It depends what you need from your body and this will change with time. One journalist who came to interview me had worked out for herself that wheat didn't really agree with her, but it wasn't such a problem that she went without it all-together. But when she was going to interview someone she would have to stop eating bread and wheat for a day or two so that her head would be clear. You may find that something similar applies to you. A pattern that suits many people is to eat difficult foods only once or twice a week at most. Or you may want to make a clean sweep, as I have done with several foods, because even small amounts give you trouble.

The Tests

The Wright Diet Food Tests are designed to give you the best possible opportunity to discover which foods and food groups suit you best, and which do not. Before you begin you must have been following stage one of the Wright Diet for at least three weeks. You will be staying on the Wright Diet of course throughout the Tests, except that you will sometimes be excluding certain foods. By the end of the Tests you will be on the way to transforming the Wright Diet into a diet more perfectly attuned to your needs than the most skilful nutritionist could ever devise for you. Your own Wright Diet.

To complete any test, stop eating everything listed under the Test for four days. Note any changes or reactions during that time and put them in your notebook. Then bring back the Test foods into your diet one by one (but don't waste time testing foods you wouldn't want to eat anyway). See the diagram below.

Food Testing

<u>WITHDRAWAL PHASE</u>   <u>RETESTING PHASE</u>

DAY 1	DAY 2	DAY 3	DAY 4	DAY 5	DAY 6	DAY 7

<u>FURTHER TESTING PHASE</u>

DAY 1	DAY 2	DAY 3	DAY 4	DAY 5	DAY 6	DAY 7

1 Each food test will last approximately two weeks.
2 You begin your withdrawal phase on Day 1 and continue to the end of Day 4.
3 During those four days you avoid every food listed under the Test, but you continue to eat other Wright Diet foods normally.

continued overleaf

Food Testing – *cont.*

4　On Day 5 you can begin retesting. By now any sensitivity to the Test foods will be at its strongest. Start to eat the Test foods you like one by one, noticing any reactions. Give yourself at least three hours before you go on to the next one, and only do so if there is no reaction.

5　If you get no reaction to a food or food group then you should include it in your own Wright Diet.

6　If you do get a reaction drink plenty of springwater and take 2–4 grams of vitamin C to help get rid of it quickly. The Test food you last ate is suspicious. Record this in your food diary, and test it again a few days later. If you get a second reaction consider removing it from your diet for a few months before testing again.

7　It is possible that you are reacting not to foods you ate today, but to something you ate yesterday. This is particularly likely if you wake up feeling awful. Retest again being more observant and allowing more time between tests.

Important If you experience severe reactions and are unable to unravel the connections with your diet, you should consult your doctor or ask to be referred to a clinical ecologist (who specialises in these reactions). See Useful Addresses on page 244.

continued opposite

Food Testing – *cont.*

If you have any reason to be concerned about your health, or if you suffer from asthma, diabetes, allergies or a disorder for which you are receiving medical attention, then you must consult your doctor before undergoing any of these tests.

Stay aware of how you feel as you eat, and watch your reactions over the next few hours. Generally, if you are going to react, it will happen within five or six hours, but it can take longer (one client noticed that she always got a migraine headache two days after eating chocolate). Record your reactions in your notebook. Don't continue with the testing process until you feel clear of the last reaction. On the whole if you get no reaction by the time the next meal is due it should be all right to test a new food.

If you get a reaction on retesting any one food you may want to check it again to make sure. Have an even larger portion the following day, or when the reaction has cleared. Once you are sure that food is a culprit you need to eliminate it for two to three months. Then, if it's a food most of us would consider healthy, try introducing it cautiously a little at a time. Do not make it a frequent part of your diet. If you find yourself having a lot of it you are addicted again and should cut it out for a longer period or for good.

Give yourself several days to reintroduce foods and be sure that all reactions have cleared before you start another Test. Do the Tests in any order that you choose.

TEST 1   Red Meat and Dairy Products

EXCLUDE THESE FOODS: Cow's milk, cow's cheese, cow's yoghurt, butter, cream, beef (e.g. steaks, hamburgers), gelatin (e.g. jelly, capsules), ox liver, veal, lard, goat's milk, yoghurt and cheese, sheep's yoghurt and cheese (e.g. feta), lamb, mutton, pork, bacon, ham, venison.

COMMENT Reactions to milk products are very common. Milk is baby food, not a natural food for adults. Many of us lose the ability to digest milk sugar (lactose) by the age of four.[54] Unless we're one of the lucky ones who retain the enzyme lactase, drinking milk after that age can cause flatulence, bloating and cramps in the lower intestines, and even diarrhoea. People with this problem, however, can usually tolerate yoghurt and cheese because the milk sugar in these has mostly been broken down by the bacteria. Milk, yoghurt and cheese can also cause other problems not necessarily connected with the milk sugar. Milk products are notoriously mucus-forming so if you suffer from catarrh, a bunged up nose or frequent colds then you should give this Test your serious attention. Milk allergy is also common (here the reaction is usually to the milk protein), perhaps because we tend to eat or drink a milk food at practically every sitting.

Milk and beef are related foods of course (although we tend to forget it), as are lamb and sheep's milk. That's why you eliminate meat and milk together. The rest of the red meats belong in this Test so that you can check out your relationship to meat as a whole. For many people this Test may be their first experience of a semi-vegetarian diet.

It's important that you exclude all sources of milk during this test. That same milk sugar, lactose, is used as an additive in the most unlikely places – even in low sodium salts and vegetable stock cubes – so check every label. And don't forget that milk and butter may be present in other foods – soups and cakes for instance.

WHAT TO EAT   For the first four days of Test 1 (see the diagram) you must strictly avoid all the foods listed above. That means basically that you don't eat red meat, milk, cheese, yoghurt or butter for that time. But there's plenty of other good food to enjoy. Try Porridge served with honey or Banana Cream; Muesli made with fruit juice; or fruit or eggs for breakfast. At lunchtime choose a grain salad like Tabbouli or a pulse dish like Humous, both served with a Green Farm Salad or Vegetable Crudités. And for dinner choose from fish, chicken, grain dishes like Buckwheat and Vegetables or one of the pulse dishes such as the Bran Feast Casserole.

TEST 2   Grains and Grain Products
EXCLUDE THESE FOODS: wheat (bread, cakes, biscuits, pastry etc.), wheat bran, wheatgerm, pasta, semolina, bulgar wheat, rye, barley, millet, corn (maize), cornflour, popcorn, corn sugar, cornstarch, oats, rice, wild rice, sugar cane, molasses, raw sugar.

Also exclude these related foods: beer, whisky, wheatgerm oil, corn oil, malt, maltose, dextrose, baker's and brewer's yeast.

COMMENT   Wheat is the second most likely food to cause difficulty, again because we overuse it (generally eating it at every meal and in between as well). The other grains may or may not be a problem, but going without any grains for a few days may be an enlightening experience for you. You will be getting a small flavour of what our diet was like for the thousands of years before grains were adopted. Be on the lookout for wheat in all sorts of foods – in sauces and as thickening, for instance.

WHAT TO EAT For the first four days of Test 2 eliminate all grains. That means no biscuits, bread, pastry, cakes, pizza or sauces made with flour. But you can eat yoghurt and banana for breakfast, or fruit or eggs. For lunch you could eat Taramasalata, Humous, baked potato or Cauliflower Cheese, served with one of the salads. And for dinner you're free to eat meat, fish, beans, nuts or cheese.

TEST 3 Eggs, 'White' Meat, and Fish
EXCLUDE THESE FOODS: Eggs, chicken, chicken liver, pheasant, duck, duck eggs, turkey, pigeon, partridge, goose, goose eggs, quail, rabbit, cod, plaice, haddock, trout, salmon, herring, mackerel, anchovy etc., crab, lobster, shrimp, prawn, oyster, mussel, squid, octopus, caviar, lumpfish caviar, other fish roe, taramasalata etc.

COMMENTS Eggs very commonly cause problems for small children. As we grow up our difficulty with eggs can be 'masked' so that we're not aware of it. Test 3 will show you how good you are at digesting eggs, and also chicken, which is another very overused food since the advent of intensive chicken farming. Fish can cause severe allergy in a few people but is generally an excellent source of protein. A mild reaction to fish might take the form of swollen tissues (water retention) or brain fogging.

WHAT TO EAT You must avoid all white meat, eggs and fish for the first four days of Test 3. But you can continue to eat red meat, dairy foods, grains, nuts and pulses. Breakfast should be no difficulty. For lunch you could have Greek Bean Salad or Cauliflower Cheese. And for dinner you could have a lamb chop, Rice and Vegetables, or Falafels (all served with salad).

TEST 4 Fruit, Nuts and Sweeteners

EXCLUDE THESE FOODS: apple, pear, banana, grape, raisin, plum, prune, pineapple, blackberry, strawberry, raspberry, gooseberry, orange, lemon, grapefruit, lime, mandarin, tangerine, plantain, date, fig, rhubarb, papaya, pomegranate, loganberry, rosehip, crabapple, loquat, quince, apricot, cherry, peach, nectarine, kumquat, lychee, mango, kiwi fruit, pawpaw, guava, blueberry, cranberry, bearberry, huckleberry, persimmon, elderberry, melon, prickly pear, mulberry etc.

Coconut, hickory, pecan, walnut, filbert, hazelnut, beechnut, chestnut, macadamia nut, brazil nut, almond, cashew, pine nut.

Honey, sugar (all kinds), molasses, date sugar, maple syrup.

Also exclude: wine, wine vinegar, brandy, champagne, juniper, gin, coconut oil.

COMMENT This Test shouldn't present too much difficulty but will help you to see how dependant you are on sweetening in your food. Use the period of the Test to get used to fuelling your blood sugar (see page 42) with complex carbohydrates such as grains, pulses and root vegetables (for instance rice, lentils, potatoes). If you get reactions from several fruit at the end of the Test you may have a salicylate problem – see Test 9.

WHAT TO EAT Don't eat fruit, nuts, wine, honey or other sweeteners for these four days. For breakfast you could eat plain yoghurt, eggs, toast or porridge without honey (which actually tastes quite good). Lunch and dinner should be no problem, but increase your salad intake if you've been used to a lot of fruit so that you don't lose alkalinity.

TEST 5 Vegetables I
EXCLUDE THESE FOODS: potato, aubergine, green pepper, red pepper, cayenne, chili, paprika, pimento, tomato, tobacco.
Cucumber, courgette (zucchini), marrow, squash, pumpkin, pumpkin seed, alfalfa, lentils, all dried beans, all sprouted beans, string beans, runner beans, beansprouts, peas, peanuts, fenugreek, carob.
Soya, soya oil, lecithin, soya milk, tofu, beancurd.
Sesame seed, sesame oil, tahini (sesame butter), linseed (flaxseed).

COMMENT The vegetables listed from potatoes to tobacco all belong to the deadly nightshade family. These foods contain solanine, a chemical known to cause such painful joints in livestock animals that graze on them, that they are sometimes found kneeling because standing is too painful. Dr Childers of the State University of New Jersey has found that 70 per cent of volunteers found some degree of relief from arthritis on a nightshade-free diet. If you suffer from arthritis do this Test very thoroughly by excluding all nightshade foods for two weeks or longer before retesting.

The pulses (lentils, peas, dried beans etc.) are superb foods for nourishing blood sugar. They're the staple diet of peasants all over the world (as a meat substitute) but we've neglected them in this country since our post-war prosperity. These foods may cause flatulence when you eat them at first, but this shouldn't necessarily be taken as a 'reaction'. This will reduce considerably as your digestive system gets used to them.

WHAT TO EAT During this Test you must go without potatoes, pulses and the listed vegetables for four days. Breakfast will be no problem. For lunch and dinner choose from fish, meat, grains and salad made with vegetables that are not part of this Test.

TEST 6 Vegetables II
EXCLUDE THESE FOODS: carrot, celery, chervil, fennel, parsley, parsnip, celeriac, coriander, sweet potato, onion, leek, spring onion, garlic, chives, asparagus, yam, beetroot, Swiss chard, spinach, olive, avocado, Chinese water chestnut, bamboo shoots, cassava, tapioca, okra (ladies' fingers).
Herbs and spices: angelica, aniseed, carraway, comfrey, cumin, dill, mint, basil, bergamot (Earl Grey), marjoram, oregano, peppermint, rosemary, sage, savory, spearmint, thyme, ginger, turmeric, cardamom, vanilla, black pepper, white pepper, nutmeg, mace, bay leaf, cinnamon, poppy seeds.
Olive oil.

COMMENT The two most common troublemakers in this section are onions and mint (and related foods – leeks, spring onions, peppermint etc.).

WHAT TO EAT Study the list and avoid these foods for four days. You shouldn't have any difficulty. Use sesame oil instead of olive oil.

TEST 7 Vegetables III
EXCLUDE THESE FOODS: lettuce, globe artichoke, jerusalem artichoke, chicory, dandelion, endive, salsify,

broccoli, brussels sprouts, cabbage, cauliflower, kale, kohlrabi, chinese cabbage, horseradish, mustard, radish, turnip, watercress, caper, burdock, chamomile, tarragon. Sunflower seeds, sunflower oil.

COMMENT   Another group of vegetables for you to test. Reactions to lettuce are not uncommon, and some people are sensitive to sunflower seeds and oil.

WHAT TO EAT   Avoiding these foods should be quite straightforward. Just consult the list before you make a salad.

TEST 8   Caffeine
EXCLUDE THE FOLLOWING: Coffee, Indian tea, China tea, Ceylon tea, coca cola, pepsi cola, chocolate, cocoa.

COMMENT   Nearly all of us are addicted to caffeine in one form or another. We use it to whip our adrenal glands into keeping us going, but we also drink it out of habit or for social reasons, and forget that it's a drug. Women with polycystic breast disease (mastitis) frequently find their symptoms disappearing when caffeine is cut out. Use the test to discover what part caffeine plays in your life.

If you are addicted withdrawal will take four days and you may get a headache in that time. But it won't be as difficult as you think, and you may discover that you can easily live without it. Don't push yourself if you really want to cut out coffee, chocolate etc. (see Part Two for how to deal with addictions).

WHAT TO EAT   There are many good drinks to try in place of tea and coffee. Try Rooibosch tea (a herb tea from health shops that tastes just like good Indian tea), or Barleycup, Pioneer or one of the other grain coffees. In place of chocolate try carob bars which you'll also find in health shops. (Don't drink decaffeinated coffee during these four days either).

TEST 9 Salicylates

EXCLUDE THESE FOODS: Cucumber, tomato.

Grapes, raisins, currants, grape juice, wine, wine vinegar, brandy, champagne.

Almonds, apples, oranges, apricots, cherries, plums, prunes, peaches, nectarines, blackberries, strawberries, raspberries, gooseberries.

Liquorice.

Potato, banana, coffee, pineapple (these four contain very little).

COMMENT 'Salicylates' are a group of foods and drinks that contain a natural form of aspirin (which is salicylic acid). Some people (including myself) get uncomfortable reactions to them. You will have covered most of these foods in other Tests. Test 9 is worth taking however if you've had reactions to any of the foods in this list, or if any of these drugs bring out a reaction: aspirin, analgesics, anti-inflammatory drugs, children's aspirin; teething, gripe water and other preparations.

WHAT TO EAT With this Test you just have to pick your way around the foods listed.

Reactions that can be caused by food	
JOINTS	pain and swelling
SKIN	itching, flushing, hives, eczema, sweating
HEAD	headache, pressure, tightness, exploding, throbbing
ENERGY	fatigue, heaviness, sleepiness
MOOD	depression, feeling negative, indifferent, crying
AROUSAL	hyperactive, silly, over-talkative, restless, anxious
MIND/SPEECH	mentally sluggish, poor concentration, memory loss, slurred speech, stammering, stuttering, spelling errors
MUSCLES	tremor, cramp, jerking, spasms, aches, stiffness
REALITY	surroundings unreal, disoriented, delusion, hallucination, suicidal
NASAL	sneezing, itching, rubbing, postnasal drip, sinus problem, stuffy feeling
THROAT & MOUTH	itching, sore, tight, swollen, hoarse
EARS	itching, blocked, tinnitis, earache, hearing loss
LUNGS & HEART	coughing, wheezing, rapid pulse, hyperventilation, chest pain, palpitations
EYES	itch, burn, black rings under, red, vision changes
DIGESTION	nausea, bloating, vomiting, cramps, diarrhoea, gall bladder problems, constant thirst
GENERAL	dizzy, lightheaded, staggering, vertigo, blackout, cold, warmth, hot flushes

PART TWO

Healing Yourself With The Wright Diet

Abundant Energy

Abundant energy, endless strength and lasting endurance. That's the dream we all have. But the reality, for most of us, falls considerably short. Most of us, in fact, suffer from chronic fatigue and just have to live our lives and make the most of it. One distinguished American physician has estimated that at least half the population is extremely tired or exhausted without knowing it.[1] For many of us fatigue has become a way of life.

On the Wright Diet that will change. Nothing has the capacity to revive weary muscles and flagging glands more than a high alkaline, high raw food diet that's packed with fuel and nutrients for cells, heart and brain. From the moment you start the change will be obvious. Especially as you throw off old stored acids and chemical poisons and your bloodstream runs clear. Stabilising your blood sugar with the first class proteins and complex carbohydrates of the Wright Diet will give you energy and purpose and a new source of strength. Gone will be that afternoon slide into slumbering incompetence. Gone will be those moments when you just can't carry on. Daily, on the Wright Diet, your energy will grow and *last* as it never has before.

But specific foods and food groups can undermine your strength too. Chronic fatigue is one of the most common signs that there may be food intolerance – with milk, cheese, eggs and grains as the most likely culprits. If you've been tired all your life then the Food Tests could help you start life again. Almost miraculously, removing the offending food from your diet can raise your energy and ability to function by anything up to 200 per cent. Cutting out milk and milk products in my own case lifted a cloud of exhaustion that holidays, early nights and acupuncture treatments had been unable to touch. When I cut milk from my diet my body responded almost overnight. Don't worry that giving up a food or drink will be a problem. Once your body has the taste of that potential, cutting out the culprit will almost be a pleasure.

ENERGY

1 Pay particular attention to keeping your blood sugar steady with complex carbohydrates and regular meals and snacks.
2 Keep your blood alkaline with plenty of fresh raw fruit and vegetables.
3 Take the Food Tests to see if any specific foods or food groups are depleting your energy.
4 Recommended supplements: the Basic Supplement Programme.

A Good Night's Sleep

You won't find a creature in the animal world that gets insomnia. Baboon or butterfly, they all have one thing in common – once every twenty-four hours they take a prolonged rest. Admittedly, some do it bolt upright. Others crawl down their burrows, or float with their fins tucked in. But they all do it. We humans on the other hand seem to have lost our rhythms. We're all trying to fit in with this nine-to-five, bed-by-midnight, set-the-alarm-clock, 'oh-my-God-I've-missed-the-train-again' routine. As a result, one in every three of us is a poor sleeper.

Before I met Brian I was quite happily semi-nocturnal. I did all my best work between ten at night and two in the morning and because I was single and self-employed this worked out fine. Provided I met my deadlines I could sleep on into the morning or take a nap in the afternoon. And when I slept, I slept. But then I met this man who liked to turn in by midnight, and to make matters worse I decided to marry him. And since it was quite obvious he wasn't going to stay up and witness my finest hour, there was nothing for it but to join him. The result was one happy marriage and one insomniac.

Over the years of nutritional searching since then I've put in a lot of hours on how to improve sleeping. Finally I managed to crack it. Now I can turn in at eleven and sleep like a log until seven. I have put together the following questionnaire to help others do the same. Using the Wright Diet you can join the well slept half of the human race.

Test Your Sleep-ability Index

1   Do your nails break easily?
2   Do you have over-sensitive emotions?
3   Are you fond of salt?
4   Do you drink coffee?
5   Do you drink alcohol in the evenings?
6   Are you fond of late night meals?
7   Are there certain foods or drinks you couldn't do without?
8   Do you find it easier to sleep during the day?

Key

1   Easily broken nails suggest a calcium deficiency, which often causes twitching muscles and restless sleep. The seeds (sunflower etc.) are a rich source of calcium and the Basic Supplement Programme should make up the rest. Check your digestion. If there's no change in your nails, you may not be absorbing your minerals properly.

2   Over-sensitive emotions are one clue to a zinc deficiency, which can also lead to unsatisfactory sleep. Add in some extra zinc for a while (between 10 and 50 mg, depending on just how sensitive you feel you are).

3   Salt can make those of us sensitive to it tense and anxious. The Wright Diet should take care of that for you.

continued opposite

Test Your Sleep-ability Index – *cont.*

4   Coffee also makes us habitually over-strung and stops us sleeping. The Wright Diet allows you one cup a day. If you take it, do it in the morning.

5   If you drink alcohol in the evening you're likely to wake up because you're thirsty and dehydrated. Remember your limited alcohol allowance on the Wright Diet. If this is still a problem, drink spring-water before bed or stop drinking in the evening.

6   Late night meals ask your stomach to digest at its lowest ebb. It wakes you up in the night and puts you off your breakfast.

7   If there are certain foods and drinks you can't do without you're addicted. There's probably a hidden food reaction that might well be keeping you awake at night. Use the Food Tests to check this out and read up the section on Cravings and Bingeing.

8   You may find this changes when you get everything else right. But if you feel your sleep rhythm needs re-educating there's a natural food supplement called tryptophan that can help this. Take 300–1000 mg each evening until you're back on rhythm. You shouldn't need it as a permanent prop.

An End To Cravings And Bingeing

Trying to change your diet when you suffer from food cravings is like trying to beat the deluge with a rowing boat. You can't do it. That's why weight loss diets almost always fail, and why there are millions of people out there struggling to resist the next chocolate bar, packet of crisps, jam scone, cream bun . . . But the level of addiction can be more serious than that. Uncontrolled food bingeing is increasingly common, especially among women. Fortunately these problems can be solved. The Wright Diet will cut through your food cravings and help you to feel human again.

Concern about heroin and serious drug abuse could make food addiction seem like a bit of a joke. After all it's hardly serious to be hooked on orange juice and it's certainly not illegal. But how soon would you go into withdrawal if the bread and jam ran out? And how long is it since your last fix of caffeine? Or perhaps you've been trying to do a cold turkey on chocolate . . . and failed?

I'm not kidding. You may not be a secret lemonade drinker, but I'm willing to bet the biggest cream cake on the trolley that you're a food addict of one kind or another. Because we all are. Every one of us. I used to be a serious salt user. I'd sprinkle it on practically everything. And even take pinches of it neat when the next meal was slow in coming. I was 'into' vinegar too. One night, staying with people I hardly knew, I sneaked into their pantry so many times that I'd finished a whole bottle of pickled onions by the morning.

You're probably completely unaware of your food addictions. Because they're likely to be the kind of food or drink you're eating every day of your life. The commonest are probably sugar, caffeine, milk and wheat because they're the ones we're most exposed to. But you can be addicted to almost anything – fruit (oranges, raisins?), meat (chicken is a common one), eggs, nuts (peanuts, peanut butter?), even vegetables (especially potatoes).

In most of us these addictions simply lead to repetitive eating patterns. For others the problem can be more serious. One woman wrote to me recently:

'I am so glad I got in touch with you because since changing to your suggested two hourly feeding regime and associated advice, my way of life and outlook has altered dramatically. When I wrote I complained of continual bingeing followed by periods of dieting accompanied by depression, hindered eyesight, severe lack of confidence, confused thinking, etc. When I received your letter I had a period of controlled eating whilst on holiday with my boyfriend and then staying with my parents, which meant regular meals were provided, but I could get snacks of whatever I wanted whenever I wanted.

'Previously this had always led to bingeing, but you're right – if you keep up your complex carbohydrate intake level and know that even when you've finished that snack you've only got two hours to go before the next one, you just don't get the awful cravings. It's now two months since I last binged and I'm feeling a bit more confident about it being a long-term cure. It is hard to believe though, after seven years of it, preceded by one and a half years of anorexia. Life is just beginning . . .

'I'm dead certain it was sugar and chocolate that were the culprits. Dairy products, wheat etc. seem to be okay. My complexion is so different and I feel so much better. I can't believe the difference in my clarity of thought and eyesight in particular. Even though I've split up with my boyfriend, I've been able to get over that okay and enjoy living now.'

The Wright Diet tackles food cravings in three ways. In the first place the alkaline input is very emotionally calming – you're far less likely to need endless cups of coffee and biscuits when you've got a good level of alkalinity in your bloodstream. Secondly it supports balanced blood sugar. Low blood sugar is probably the major trigger to most bouts of bingeing. And thirdly it helps you to identify the specific foods to which your body is intolerant – curiously you're most likely to be addicted to the very foods your body can't actually handle.

Food addiction, like all other types, seems to work by the hair of the dog principle. If you eat a food that hits your system hard you get a hangover. The quickest way out of feeling dreadful is to get another hit. You reach for the same food again and pretty soon you're addicted. The Food Tests will help you to identify the culprits, then all you have to do is allow the diet to support you until you feel strong enough to lose them from your diet one by one. I've had a lot of success helping people to do this. What most people tell me is that once the diet takes hold they either find they can take their chocolate or leave it (or their bread, biscuits, salted crisps or whatever it is), or they simply don't want to touch that food anyway, and that it's easy.

IF YOU SUFFER FROM FOOD CRAVINGS

1 Follow the diet carefully, making sure you have a sustaining snack every two hours, with emphasis on the complex carbohydrates – whole grains (oats, rye, wheat, etc.), pulses (lentils), root vegetables (e.g. potatoes), and fruit (bananas, apples).

2 Maintain your alkalinity at all times. If you start to feel acidified eat some fresh fruit.

3 Identify any specific addictions using the Food Tests and try to keep clear of them, at least until you feel you have the problem under control.

4 If you do start to binge you can help to stop it by drinking at least one pint of good springwater, and eating fresh fruit.

5 Don't make the mistake of trying to cut down on food in order to lose weight. Get your cravings under control and your weight will begin to take care of itself.

6 Recommended Supplements: the Basic Supplement Programme (see page 231).

Losing Weight

There is only one real way to lose weight, and that is to do it naturally. Gimmicks, crash diets and desperate efforts may lead to short-lived triumphs. But hard-lost pounds always sneak back, and you have to start again. So up and down goes your weight in an inevitable cycle of diet-binge-and-diet-again. This may be hard on your wardrobe, but it's even harder on your body.

Losing weight on the Wright Diet is a totally different experience. You need never suffer hunger, guilt or defeat again – because this diet works with your nature and not against it. The Wright Diet brings back long-buried instincts that help you regain the balance destroyed by your earlier eating patterns. On this diet you adjust without effort to your real needs for food. Under all those layers there is a natural you with a natural weight. Getting back to that weight on the Wright Diet will actually be a pleasure.

The Wright Diet will help you to

- lose those cravings and forget about bingeing
- eat less without ever getting hungry
- encourage your body to burn (and not store) your food as fat
- lose that excess fluid that's been waterlogging your tissues
- discover foods in your diet that have been stopping you lose weight

Being overweight is a modern disease. It was first noticed in England in the late eighteenth century. Even in the

1930s it was still rare enough in Africa to be remarked on. Among primitive people all over the world both men and women stayed slim and their weight actually tended to fall after the age of 30.[2]

Zulu women living in the traditional way in the 1950s for instance had an average weight of 8½ stone by the age of 30. But Zulu women who moved away from their villages and took up a Western lifestyle in the city actually managed to grow 50 lb heavier than their country sisters within twenty years.[2]

Once you've seen the evidence, there are no prizes for guessing what causes weight gain. All over the world, when primitive people start eating sugar and refined flour, cutting out the fibre, stepping up the fat and adding chemicals – they get fat.

Can you imagine stone-age cavewoman sweating over how many calories there are to a dinosaur? Of course not. That cavewoman stayed slim without having to think about it. Nor does it make sense to count the calories of the foods that people eat today. Because most of these foods, especially those made from sugar or refined flours, *are actually the cause of the problem itself*. That's why it's so hard to lose weight on conventional diets. On most diets you just eat less of these very same foods. But on the Wright Diet you switch to real foods – the kind we've all been eating for thousands of years without getting fat.

On the Wright Diet you forget about calories and start to listen to your body. Then and only then can you shed the pounds, and never put them back again.

Eating Less by Eating More Often

The major imbalance that causes weight gain is almost certainly irregular blood sugar. Every time your blood sugar peaks and falls back down again, you feel hungry.

If you have a blood sugar problem this can happen several times a day. You get hungry but your body doesn't really need more food.

Any sugar-based foods can set the ball rolling. Biscuits, sweets, cakes, and soft drinks, for instance – full of the sugar we were never really designed to eat. Your blood sugar rises swiftly when you eat these foods. Your body responds by pumping out the hormone insulin. Blood sugar falls again but far too quickly (see page 42). Very soon you're desperate for more to eat. On a cycle like this you can eat two or three thousand calories a day on top of what you really need.

The Wright Diet cuts through those cycles right away, and stabilises your blood sugar. It feeds you bulky natural foods that give you a steady rise in blood sugar, and avoids those sudden peaks and troughs. With steady blood sugar you only get hungry when it's really time to eat. On the Wright Diet you can eat less without getting hungry and actually enjoy losing weight.

Timing is important too. Those morning and afternoon snacks built into the Wright Diet needn't be large. But they're there to keep your blood sugar stable. Even if you're trying to lose weight you should only cut them out when you really don't need them. Forget those ideas about starving until the evening and then letting rip. Five or six small meals a day can help you sustain such an even blood sugar that you actually eat less by eating more frequently.

Turning Up Your Metabolism
For years fatties have been trying to blame their metabolism. Now science has come up with a theory that could make them feel justified. It concerns a rather unusual feature of the body called the brown fat. When the body

burns off excess food (rather than turning it into fat), it is the brown fat cells that are responsible. Brown fat cells are packed with tiny biochemical furnaces. When they're stimulated the excess food we eat is turned into heat, and we don't put on weight. And some of us are better at it than others.

The message that tells the brown fat to do this comes from the thyroid gland – the gland at the base of the neck which controls metabolic rate (how fast or how slow we tick over.) It used to be thought that people whose brown fat was underfunctioning (and who consequently gained weight) had poor thyroid function. But it now looks as if it's the conversion of these thyroid hormones into their active form that causes the problem.[3]

The Wright Diet will bring your brown fat to peak activity to help you lose weight and keep it off. Research now shows that the kind of diet which favours brown fat metabolism is one that is high in complex carbohydrates (vegetables, grains and pulses), medium in protein and low in fat[4] – in fact the Wright Diet. Diets that are too high in protein or fat can actually 'poison' brown fat and reduce its fat burning ability.[5]

It has even been shown that vegetable oils are more effective in activating brown fat than animal fats or partially hydrogenated vegetable oils (such as polyunsaturated margarines[6]), and that natural sugars such as those found in fruit promote more brown cell activity than refined sugars.[7] To make sure that the thyroid gland is getting enough raw material for its hormones you also need plenty of fish or seaweed for iodine. B vitamins are important too, and so are zinc and copper. So all your brown fat needs are well covered by the Wright Diet and the Basic Supplement Programme.

The Water Factor

Several years ago one of the newspapers carried a story about a medical diet, with a rather surprising side effect, that was being used in a special heart clinic in America. The side effect was that people who went to the clinic for heart treatment were also losing a lot of weight! Not surprisingly the clinic had become highly successful. Whether they had heart trouble or not people were checking in just to get the benefits of the diet.

The diet itself was very monotonous – just rice and fruit. What was really interesting was the nature of the weight loss itself. Fruit and rice add up to a diet high in potassium, the mineral needed to balance the water-retaining mineral sodium. And the weight loss (in some cases consisting of several stone) was principally a loss of water not of fat (people suffering from water retention have plump, waterlogged body tissues that are easily mistaken for fat).

Diets that promote water loss are often regarded as ineffective. You lose water on the diet, the critics say, but afterwards it all goes back on again. Not so. At least not on the Wright Diet. The secret is to find the cause of the imbalance. When you correct this, the water stays away.

People who have lived for years on a high salt diet are likely to have an excess of sodium in their bodies, and a deficiency of the mineral that counterbalances it, potassium. The combination of high sodium and low potassium can lead to water retention. The Wright Diet is high in potassium and low in sodium, so you correct this imbalance and lose your excess water.

Foods That Cause Weight Gain

But a sodium/potassium imbalance isn't the only cause of water retention. Any food to which you're sensitive can cause it too. The most dramatic case I ever saw of this was one of our own research assistants. During a consultation about her general health I recommended that she try the first Wright Diet Food Test – excluding dairy products and red meat. A week later she walked into my office astonishingly different. Without setting out to lose weight she had actually lost about five pounds, which was interesting but not remarkable. What was impressive was her shape. Gone was her chubby rounded figure. In its place was a svelte, streamlined and *thin* young woman. She had lost weight, but even more dramatically she had lost inches. Her face, her body, her legs – in fact every part of her – had shed its puppy fat, and her eyes were sparkling too.

Since then I've seen this transformation many times. This form of water retention is known as allergic oedema,[8] but that simply means that food to which you're sensitive may cause you to put on weight, most of which is water. If you're one of those people who just can't lose weight on conventional diets then this may be your problem. If you suffer from allergic oedema you can put on up to a stone in weight after a single meal. Some women bloat so badly after meals that they look six months pregnant. These are extreme reactions however. Most people with this problem are simply carrying somewhere between two and eight pounds excess weight as water all the time.

In our research assistant's case, it was milk that had caused her fluid retention. Milk and cheese are common triggers with this kind of weight problem, but wheat, yeast, eggs and other foods can cause it too. If you have a tendency to bloating or water retention, work through the Food Tests and find your own culprits – when you get it right you could have a lot less to lose!

Not The Usual Diet Formula

The Wright Diet approach to weight loss may seem strange if you are used to thinking only in terms of calories. Of course quantity counts, but this diet looks behind the obvious to find out why you have gained weight in the first place.

By balancing your blood sugar so that you are not constantly over-eating, by fuelling your brown fat with foods that promote metabolism, by eliminating salt so that you don't carry extra pounds of fluid, and by finding out which foods specifically promote this fluid weight gain, you will develop a way of eating that allows you to eat to satisfaction while actually losing weight.

Your rate of weight loss may be rapid, but it is more likely to be slow and steady. Don't be anxious about it. If you're concerned only to lose weight as quickly as possible you should remember that rapid weight loss through extreme methods generally only leads to rapid weight gain soon after. You are aiming for the root causes of your problem. Once you know those you will be able to keep your weight down for life.

A word of caution – the Wright Diet will reduce you to your natural weight, and no further. It can't help you reach those semi-anorexic states of starvation that some women think are attractive. If you're 5 feet 5 inches tall for instance, your natural weight is somewhere between eight and nine stone. Accept that your body has its own natural weight, the one at which it is naturally streamlined and ready for action. It is this healthy weight that the Wright Diet will help you to reach.

TO LOSE WEIGHT

1 Bring your blood sugar under control with three small-ish meals and two to three snacks in between, all on Wright Diet foods – high in vegetables, complex carbohydrates, fruit, fish and white meat.

2 Be very careful to keep your food low in salt, and eat lots of fresh fruit and vegetables to keep your potassium intake high.

3 Eat plenty of seaweed (for iodine) with your meals. You can get powdered kelp for sprinkling, or use it as shown in the recipes.

4 Take the Food Tests to check whether there are foods that prevent you losing weight.

5 You can increase your weekly Fast Days to two if you wish, either consecutively or apart. On your Fast Days eat lots of fruit and fresh raw vegetables and drink plenty of natural juices.

6 Recommended supplements: the Basic Supplement Programme.

Premenstrual Blues Away

I can remember standing in the school lunch queue when I was sixteen and wanting to throttle the girl just in front of me. What the poor girl had done, if anything, I have no idea. But I do know that this was the first time it dawned on me that it was always around *that* time of the month that I seemed to lose all semblance of equanimity and turn into something more closely resembling a she-wolf.

We called it the 'curse' in those days. And it did seem like that. Whether or not we experienced a premenstrual build-up (no one talked about such things at the time), we all suffered from painful cramps and varying degrees of disability. It never occurred to us that this state of affairs was anything other than 'normal'. But I now know that women don't have to suffer like this. There's nothing normal about it at all.

As soon as I began work on the Wright Diet my PMT days began to evaporate. Later the cramps went too. Nowadays I *enjoy* the first day of my period. It's a day when I feel contemplative and inclined to gaze out of windows contentedly. Sometimes. I feel slightly vulnerable in a rather pleasant way, and very female. If you do suffer from the premenstrual syndrome (irritability, water retention, cravings, depression), or other period problems such as painful cramps, the Wright Diet will be your first step towards real normality.

Diet Helps PMT
Recently a list of dietary changes that have so far been found to help the symptoms of PMT was quoted in the

Journal of Reproductive Medicine. You'll notice that every one of these suggestions is already contained within the guidelines of the Wright Diet Stage One:

- Limit consumption of refined sugar, salt, red meat, alcohol, coffee, tea and chocolate.
- Limit intake of protein to 1gm/kg of body weight/day.
- Limit intake of dairy products.
- Limit intake of fats, mainly saturated and cooked.
- Increase intake of complex carbohydrates.
- Increase intake of green leafy vegetables, legumes, whole grains and cereals.
- Increase intake of foods containing linolenic acid (sunflower seeds, linseeds etc.).[9]

Each of these dietary changes helps prevent the premenstrual syndrome in a specific way, and is based on sound theory or has been demonstrated in scientific trials. For instance, women who suffer from tension and irritability before their periods have sometimes been found to be consuming much higher levels of dairy products than women who are free of symptoms.[10] Dr Guy Abraham who has been working on nutritional therapy for women sufferers for a number of years believes that excess intake of calcium from dairy products may interfere with energy supplies to the brain,[9] triggering episodes of discomfort and potential aggression.

A high sugar intake on the other hand may set the scene for premenstrual cravings – a strong desire for sweets and chocolates in the days leading up to menstruation. Paradoxically, a high level of sugar in the diet can make the body cells more sensitive to insulin, the hormone that lowers blood sugar.[11] So eating a lot of sugar can lead to *low* blood sugar which is precisely what may trigger a bout of cravings. And it seems that this effect may be amplified in the second half of the female cycle,[12] making premenstrual cravings especially common among women who eat too much sugar in their diets.

Each of the dietary changes listed above has similarly been found to trigger one or more of the symptoms that make up the premenstrual syndrome. So following the Wright Diet is likely to make a significant difference to all your premenstrual problems. The diet will also help with period pains and cramps. Other difficulties such as irregularity and heavy bleeding may sort themselves out too (especially in conjunction with the supplements given below).

Vitamins and Minerals for Period Problems
There are also nutritional supplements which can help, specifically vitamin B6 (backed up by the whole B Complex), magnesium, vitamin C, vitamin E and zinc. For most women the Basic Supplement Programme should provide enough of each of these nutrients. But extra vitamin B6 and magnesium may be called for (a maximum 200 mg of each should be sufficient). For oversensitivity and depression we find extra zinc (up to 50 mg elemental) very helpful.

In the last few years it has been found that prostaglandins (hormone-like chemicals found throughout the body) may play a part in the premenstrual syndrome, and in cramping. The good guys, certain prostaglandins that inhibit others that trigger pain and inflammation, are made from a body chemical called gamma linolenic acid, or GLA. Our bodies make GLA from the linoleic acid in our food (plentiful in seeds like sunflower and sesame).

But for our bodies to make sufficient GLA to keep us free from PMT and period problems we need a good supply of the nutrients listed above (the B vitamins, particularly B3 and B6, vitamin C, magnesium and zinc). The Wright Diet and Basic Supplement Programme should provide enough of these nutrients, but be particularly conscious of getting sufficient good oils by eating seeds such as linseeds, sunflower seeds, pumpkin seeds and sesame.

Evening Primrose Oil which contains about 8 per cent GLA can provide you with a short cut if you're not making enough of your own, but it's important to get your diet and Basic Supplements right before you resort to this.

FREEDOM FROM PMT

1 Check the list of dietary changes at the beginning of the section and modify your diet accordingly, especially keeping your dairy intake low.

2 Keep your blood sugar in balance, particularly in the second half of your cycle with small fruit and complex carbohydrate snacks.

3 Include plenty of seeds in your diet – sunflower, sesame, pumpkin, linseed.

4 Recommended supplements:
The Basic Supplement Programme
plus (if you feel you need extra help):
vitamin B6 50–200 mg,
magnesium 100–200 mg (elemental – chelate, orotate or ascorbate are best),
zinc up to 50 mg (elemental – chelate or orotate are best),
Evening Primrose Oil 250–1000 mg

Breast Swelling and Cysts

Many women experience breast swelling in the days before menstruation, but some develop cysts that can be very painful, although not life-threatening. (These cysts do however increase your risk of breast cancer.) The condition is called fibrocystic breast disease, or sometimes cystic mastitis. The Wright Diet Stage One should help women suffering from painful breasts, especially in conjunction with the supplements recommended for PMT. But the real benefits may come when you take Test 8 – for caffeine.

Several years ago an American physician, Dr J. P. Minton, made headlines in medical journals with the claim that breast cysts could be prevented on a caffeine-free diet.[13] Of 20 women who had followed his advice, 13 lost all symptoms within six months and another 3 within 1½ years. Age, Dr Minton finds, is an important factor. Younger women are cured comparatively quickly, whereas one woman, a 66-year-old college professor with very severe mastitis, didn't respond completely for two years, but her breasts today are normal. We've been passing on this advice with good results too. One Green Farm member with cysts arranged with her doctor for a six-month stay of surgery while she changed her diet and cut out coffee, tea and chocolate. When the six months were up her breasts were trouble-free.

If you have trouble with your breasts use the period of the Wright Diet Stage One to help you reduce your caffeine intake. Remember you don't have to fight yourself to shed an addiction. Start by building yourself up with good food and the Basic Supplement Programme, then take Test 8. You may get a headache for a day or two, but you'll be clear of addiction at the end of four days. If you can manage it, cut out all sources of caffeine for two whole weeks before your next period is due, and see if your breasts are any different at the 'worst' time (usually the day before the period begins). Whether or not you notice any change in such a short time, you'd be well advised to go 'caffeine-free' if you suffer from cystic mastitis[14] (see the recipe section for good alternatives).

Several vitamins and minerals have been found to help too. Vitamin E on its own has helped regress painful breast cysts.[15] In a recent study sponsored by the American Cancer Society, Dr Robert London gave 26 women 600 international units of vitamin E a day in a double blind trial. Within eight weeks 10 of the women had lost their symptoms completely, and another 12 were 'fair responders'.[16] If you're going to try vitamin E therapy however, you should check that you don't have high blood pressure.

In addition to the Basic Supplement Programme you may need extra vitamin B6 and magnesium, to the same level as with period problems. Iodine has also been found to help in some cases, so remember to bring those seaweeds into your diet (see recipe section). Finally, check with your doctor if you think you may have benign breast cysts.

FOR BENIGN BREAST CYSTS

1 Follow the Wright Diet as indicated for PMT.
2 Take Test 8 (for caffeine) if possible giving yourself two caffeine-free weeks before your next period.
3 Eat plenty of seaweeds.
4 Recommended supplements: the Basic Supplement Programme plus up to 500 i.u. of vitamin E (check with your doctor that you don't have high blood pressure).

Radiant Skin And Shining Hair

If I had to select one aspect of my health to attribute to the Wright Diet, it would be the remarkable response of my skin. I know, of course, that clear and healthy skin reflects the health of my whole body, but I'm also vain and old enough to enjoy the constant compliments. If you suffer from pasty, dull or spotty skin, take heart. The Wright Diet will clear your spots and toxins, and leave you glowing. In six months your friends will be telling you you look ten years younger.

Just cutting all that 'junk' from your diet will give your skin a new beginning. When your diet is full of rubbish – sugar, refined flour, fried foods and chemical additives – a lot of the wastes that the body can't eliminate are dumped in the skin. The skin after all is an organ of elimination; it's sometimes called the 'third kidney'. And when the liver, kidneys and colon are overloaded, the skin has to take on a lot of the work. Eventually the skin itself gets blocked. Then toxins build up in the tissues attracting spots and infection, and promoting pasty and unhealthy skin.

But when you begin the Wright Diet your skin will start a cleansing process almost immediately. The high alkalinity will revive those tired and flagging tissues. The vitamin-packed raw salads will encourage fresh growth and healing. Skin-nourishing foods such as fruit, seeds and seaweeds will bring exciting changes in moisture and texture, and the Basic Supplement Programme will encourage new life right down where the skin cells are forming.

Healing Troubled Skin

Cleansing the body is even more important if you have a difficult skin condition. One herbal formula we have found that helps to cleanse the skin from the inside is a combination of equal parts of dandelion, burdock, sarsaparilla and yellow dock. Taken as tea, or in a tablet, these four herbs seem to be able to unblock channels of elimination through kidneys, liver, colon, and skin and to bring about a cleansing that helps the skin to clear and repair itself. If you're impatient to see the cleansing miracle try the Fast Day Menu on page 105. Infections, blemishes and patches of rough or dry skin will heal and vanish in double quick time. Even the easiest level of fasting will start to soften and clear your skin within days.

Troubled skin however may need extra supplements too. If you suffer from acne, eczema, dermatitis or psoriasis, for instance, you will need to boost your diet with vitamin A, zinc, the B vitamins (especially vitamin B6) and the essential fatty acids (which come from the seeds). Shredding lots of carrots into your salads is one of the best ways to increase your vitamin A. But you may also want to top up your Basic Supplement Programme with an extra 25,000 i.u. of beta-carotene (a non-toxic supplement which the body can convert into vitamin A), and up to 50 mg of zinc.

For most skin problems I recommend an extra 100 mg of vitamin B6, and of course, the seeds – sesame, sunflower, pumpkin and linseed – will help to clear your skin too. Also, for difficult conditions, vitamin B5 (up to 1 g) and two or three extra grams of vitamin C will help your body to make its own natural cortisone.

You may find you get faster results on a higher intake of beta-carotene or vitamin A (which is usually from fish oil), especially with acne and psoriasis. The evidence so far is that you can safely take up to 50,000 i.u. of vitamin A (which is the level Dr Weston Price found commonly being consumed by primitive people), but it's best if you do this under supervision. So far there is no evidence of toxicity with beta-carotene.

But if you're impatient to see what the Wright Diet miracle can do for your skin, start taking the Food Tests as soon as you can. Your acne may be triggered by chocolate for instance, and eczema can be caused by a masked intolerance of egg. Once you discover which foods do and don't work for you, your eczema (or any other skin condition) may simply melt away.

The Wright Diet Will Help Your Hair Too
Much of what works for skin is good for hair too. Our hair, after all, is made from specialised skin cells. On the Wright Diet your hair will gleam, and grow faster. Split ends and dandruff will vanish, and within months your hair will be thicker and stronger and richer in colour. Soon your hairdresser and even your friends will be noticing the difference.

In the first place a shining mane needs food. Not just good food, but very good food. Hair isn't essential to your survival, remember. In terms of your body's priorities, hair is low on the list. So getting the nourishment to the roots of your hair means feeding the rest of you very well too. Two of the best foods for hair are fish and seaweeds. Both are rich in iodine and the trace minerals which are so often scarce in foods grown on land. (Think of the Japanese. They have exceptionally strong and healthy hair which often keeps its colour into old age – and the Japanese eat a lot of seafoods.) All seafoods are rich in iodine and other trace minerals which are often scarce in foods grown on land. Iodine is needed for the healthy function of the thyroid gland, which is absolutely essential to healthy hair and skin. The seeds (sunflower etc.) are needed here too, especially if you have dandruff or scalp problems.

The Basic Supplement Programme will give you a lot of the extra nutrients you need for improving your hair. The minerals and the B vitamins are particularly important. If you feel your need is greater because of thinning or poor quality locks you can safely double the mineral dosage, and take five or six kelp tablets for extra trace minerals. Thinning hair however is a message from the body. It may be telling you that your diet has been inadequate, but it could also be a sign that your digestion is inefficient. If you're aware of any digestive discomfort, try a course of digestive enzymes.

FOR CLEAR AND BEAUTIFUL SKIN

1 A high alkaline diet full of fresh vegetables and fruit.
2 Include the seeds in your diet.
3 Fast regularly on fresh fruit, vegetables, and juices (once a week is sufficient).
4 Check with the Food Tests that there is no specific food or food group causing skin problems.
5 Recommended supplements:
   The Basic Supplement Programme
   plus (if you need them)
   beta-carotene 25,000 i.u.
   zinc up to 50 mg (elemental, best forms are chelate or orotate)
   vitamin B6 up to 100 mg
   vitamin B5 up to 1 g
   vitamin C up to 3 g
   (It's best to add these extra supplements in one at a time so that you can tell whether they are helpful or not.)

FOR A HEAD OF HEALTHY HAIR

1   Eat plenty of fish and seaweed for iodine and trace minerals.
2   Include plenty of the seeds in your diet for essential fatty acids.
3   A course of digestive enzymes (from good health food shops) could help to improve this. Use the Food Tests to see if you can improve your digestion. It could help you keep your hair on.
4   Recommended supplements:
    The Basic Supplement Programme
    plus (if you need it)
    1 extra multivitamin
    Kelp tablets, up to 6

Goodbye To Anxiety And Depression

I know very well what it is to feel a cloud hanging over you. I spent a good part of my younger days feeling dreadful, which is probably why I became a psychologist. During my various trainings I learned a lot of techniques and exercises that were very helpful, for myself and later for my clients. But nothing stopped me falling into the trough again, even though I did have the techniques to haul myself out. Now I know why.

As a psychologist who really used to believe that person-to-person talking, along with certain physical therapies (such as osteopathy), were the only ways to clear up anxiety and depression, I was humbled by the power of nutrition when I finally experienced it. After years of trying to keep my balance on nothing but shifting sands, the first high-alkaline diet I was given was like a life-raft from heaven. Within weeks I felt strong and stable in a way that I never had before. Problems still came to me of course but they were solvable. From my new base of strength and stability there was no obstacle I couldn't jump. That was why I gave up psychology and began to work with nutrition.

You can have this balance and freedom too when you start the Wright Diet. I don't mean that you'll never feel sad or stressed again. Of course not. But you will bounce back quickly. And as time goes on, and the cleansing and healing process of the diet gets to work on you, you'll start to find an inner strength and maturity that you never thought possible. I know this because I've seen it in myself and in countless Green Farm members over the years. The diet will cut through the nonsense and let you find the real you. I don't mean of course that you won't need to get to know yourself better, or to heal your body with good physical therapies. Just that your diet underpins both of these, and neither can really work well until you get it right.

The Wright Diet Changes Your Mood

In reality it isn't so much what the Wright Diet does as what it doesn't do, that brings about the miracle. Peeling away those layers of sugar-snacks, deep-fried dinners, acid toxins, chemical residues and general junk food is only the first important step in the freeing of your spirit. Raising your alkalinity with a high raw vegetable diet, and balancing your blood sugar with complex carbohydrates and an understanding of your energy needs, must come next. Finally, tuning your diet with the Food Tests and discovering the right diet for you will help to rebalance your chemistry and strengthen your nervous system until humour, courage and optimism are part of your everyday life.

Depression can range from deep and despairing to just feeling down. Whatever the intensity, the mistake we all make is to think that it's something 'out there' that causes it. Whatever's happening in our lives, the depression itself is created inside. Lift the depression and you'll cope with life, whatever it's throwing at you. So put aside your problems and get into the Diet. Work at really alkalising your blood and balancing your blood sugar. That alone, along with the Basic Supplement Programme, should lift your mood on a permanent basis.

But if you still feel a problem, press on to the Food Tests. Some of your everyday foods may be triggering depression even though you don't suspect it. I've come across several people who were depressed by wheat (bread, pasta, biscuits etc.), and many more who couldn't handle chocolate without falling into despair. Your own reactions might be quite different of course.

Anxiety, if anything, can be even more gripping when it's got its teeth into you. We're all masters at running in ever-decreasing circles trying to control what we believe is bothering us. Alas, it never works, because this state of anxiety is also internal; and no amount of external huffing and puffing will really pacify it. Once again you need to work on alkalinity and balancing blood sugar. Nothing makes you grumpier than an over-acid diet, and low blood sugar itself frequently sets off anxiety and panic. Actual anxiety or panic attacks however may call for Food Tests again. One client had her first real panic attack after eating rather a lot of cheese. Another found his anxiety rose with his consumption of peanut butter sandwiches!

Certain vitamins and minerals are important here too. The key vitamins for both anxiety and depression are the B complex, which help to calm and smooth the running of the nervous system. Vitamin C is also essential to help detoxify the blood and help make anti-stress hormones. Among minerals calcium, and even more particularly magnesium, are calming and strengthening. For all of these the Basic Supplement Programme should be sufficient. But the missing key, I often find, is zinc.

I was once asked, when I visited the office of a magazine for which I was going to do some writing, if there was anything I could suggest for one of the staff who was so depressed that no one felt they could help her. There was nowhere we could talk privately so I suggested that she call me. The next day she described how sad and lonely she felt, and answered a lot of questions over the phone.

I suggested some changes along the lines of the Wright Diet (particularly to balance blood sugar) and just three supplements to try until we could meet and talk in more depth – a good B complex, a calcium with magnesium tablet, and 50 mg of zinc.

Three weeks later I was back at the magazine. 'Have you seen her?' they all asked, and then she came bounding in. She didn't have to say anything; she was a completely different girl. In her case nothing more was needed. I heard from her and her mother over the next year or two. She stayed positive and healthy on simple changes of diet and just those three extra supplements.

FREEDOM FROM ANXIETY AND DEPRESSION

1   A high alkaline diet with plenty of fresh vegetables and fruit.
2   Regular fruit and vegetable fasting without letting yourself get hungry.
3   Support your blood sugar with good complex carbohydrates (see the recipes starting on page 187).
4   Take the Food Tests. Something you are eating may well be making you depressed or anxious.
5   Recommended supplements:
    The Basic Supplement Programme
    plus
    zinc, up to 50 mg (elemental – as chelate or orotate).

Coming Off Tranquillizers

Quitting tranquillizers doesn't have to be the grim cold turkey affair that some people experience. In the first place you have to admit that you're hooked and really want to stop. But once you've crossed that hurdle the Wright Diet will give you all the support you need to make a smooth transition back to normality.

The problem for most people when they come off the drug is that they have to cope with the original state of anxiety, and on top of that with a body which has now been further depleted by the drug itself. This can make the first few months after quitting a tranquillizer very grim indeed. Not surprisingly only the very courageous attempt it. But there is another way. Using the Wright Diet you work at it from both ends. Start by taking the right direction as outlined from page 99, and the Basic Supplement Programme to build yourself up. Take it gently. Pay special attention to keeping your blood sugar steady. Remember to take your Feast Days, and don't take more than one Fast Day at a time.

As you start to feel stronger reduce your tranquillizer by about 15 per cent (in consultation with your doctor of course). Don't be over-ambitious. Just cut it down a little at a time, and don't be afraid to increase it again if you panic. The whole process might take several months, depending on how long you've been hooked. Double your Basic Supplement Programme for at least two weeks before you take the last step, and continue at that level until you're stable again. Over the whole of this period you may need to increase your vitamin C. This seems to help with all addictions. An upper limit of five or six grams should be completely non-toxic (if this dose causes loosening of the bowel simply reduce it).

COMING OFF TRANQUILLIZERS

1   Keep your blood sugar strong with regular snacks and meals.
2   Double the Basic Supplement Programme for 2 weeks before cutting down your tranquillizer.
3   Vitamin C, up to 6 g.

Energy For Sports

When a 61-year-old Australian amateur beat 11 international runners and knocked two days off the record for the Sydney to Melbourne run a few years ago the whole world was forced to sit up and take notice.[17] Perhaps it was to do with his diet, they all said. Cliff Young claimed to be an avid consumer of potatoes and pumpkins. Was this the discovery of pumpkin power?

Having the energy to run a race is definitely an art. The television advertisements and several sports nutrition companies promote concentrated glucose, usually in the form of a drink. Glucose gives a surge of energy all right. But what it gives, it also takes away. Almost any form of sugar, and particularly glucose, will give raised energy for about 20 or 30 minutes. But eating sugar almost always triggers low blood sugar. Within an hour of that glucose drink you'll be losing concentration and flagging.

Many of these drinks are also laced with salt. Salt hits the adrenal glands, raising blood sugar hormonally, eventually tapping into the same cycle as the sugar. And not only will salt also sap your energy, it may raise your blood pressure too. Hardly the way to keep going through a normal day, and certainly not the way to run a marathon.

The number one key to energy is always the same, and Cliff Young's secret was, I believe, none other than this; for 61 years he'd lived on a diet that really supported his blood sugar. His favourite meal of boiled potatoes, greens and mashed pumpkins was Cliff Young's own perfect combination of complex carbohydrates. He took up running at the age of 57 but his diet had been nourishing his blood sugar for a lifetime. And that counted for more, against international runners, than youth.

In recent years a system of carbohydrate loading has become popular among runners and serious athletes. It entails starving and then loading the body with carbohydrate in the days leading up to a race.

The form of carbohydrate usually suggested, pasta, couldn't be more counter-productive. All wheat, but particularly the kind used to make pasta, is high in gluten, a sticky protein that can slow the passage of food by several days.

If running a marathon full of half-digested pasta isn't wise, the principle of training on a diet of complex carbohydrates is. Cliff Young has shown us that. Optimum energy for active sports, however, calls for more than eating carbohydrates for the last four or five days before an event. Any sportsman or woman who wants the best from their body must learn to sustain their blood sugar almost permanently. You don't have to eat pumpkin or even boiled potato. You just have to find the combination of protein, carbohydrate foods and fresh vegetables to make this possible. There is no better way to do this than with the Wright Diet.

ENERGY FOR SPORTS

1 A high complex carbohydrate diet to support your blood sugar (see the recipes and try the pulse recipes in particular).

2 Avoid all sugared and salted sports drinks.

3 Recommended supplements:
   The Basic Supplement Programme
   plus (if you wish)
   vitamin E, up to 1000 i.u. (but check with your doctor)
   kelp, up to 6 tablets
   vitamins B5, up to 1000 mg (for adrenal energy).

Life Without Headaches

I've suffered from headaches all my life. Not migraines, admittedly, but infuriating pains and tensions bad enough to make sure I was never at my best. Headaches hurt, there's no doubt about that. At their worst they can be totally disabling. But even the mild ones can hamper your functioning and ruin your day. If you take a painkiller, you're still suffering at a deeper level – you haven't removed the cause. Yet without drugs the pain could last for hours or even days.

For me, knowing that I need never get another headache is like feeling free to be myself for the first time in my life. If you are a headache sufferer you can use the Wright Diet to get the same freedom for yourself.

Surprisingly, the most common cause of headaches is almost certainly low blood sugar (see page 42). That drop in the blood sugar finds your weakness, whatever it is. Some of us get snappy and go looking for an argument; some of us feel exhausted and start to slow down; some of us get cravings that can turn into addictions. And a lot of us get headaches. So when you start the Wright Diet, and begin to balance your blood sugar, you could be pain-free for the first time in your life. This is particularly true if the attacks always come at the same time of the day. The answer to your problem could be as simple as making sure you're well enough fed.

But if the first stage of the Wright Diet doesn't leave you headache-free, you must go on to the Food Tests. Specific foods are the second most likely triggers to your pain. The classic ones, of course, are foods like chocolate, red wine and cheese, but you shouldn't assume that they will be the answer for you. Chocolate gives me spots, not a headache, for instance. But a cucumber puts me in purgatory for hours. So work your way through the Food Tests carefully. Remember that you may actually get a headache in the first two days of withdrawal from one of the food groups. This is actually a sign that one or more of those foods may be causing you trouble. But you'll only know for sure when you eat the food again and get a headache (this may happen immediately or be delayed for a number of hours).

Niacin, one of the B vitamins, can help stave off a headache by dilating the blood vessels in the head. To do this you need to take 50–100 mg of niacin as the headache starts, in addition to the Basic Supplement Programme. Niacin, however, brings out a flush all over your skin, so you have to be prepared to go rather red in the face for half an hour or so. But it's quite safe. In fact it's beneficial. It promotes blood sugar balance and good circulation, and can help you feel more emotionally secure too. The calcium and magnesium in the multimineral formula will help too.

Finally if the headaches continue to be bad you should have your head and spine checked by a good cranial osteopath. Compression of bones in the skull or of vertebrae can exacerbate headaches or even cause them, and this can often be released quite simply.

FREEDOM FROM HEADACHES

1 Balance your blood sugar with the Wright Diet.
2 Take the Food Tests to see if certain foods are causing your headaches.
3 Recommended supplements:
   The Basic Supplement Programme
   plus
   vitamin B3 (niacin), 50–100 mg (remember this can cause flushing).

PART THREE
The Right Food

Basic Food Types

The foods that you should eat on the Wright Diet fall into two groups.

Class One foods are those that will give you high level health and energy. You should eat these freely unless you discover from the Food Tests that some of them are not for you.

Class Two foods are those that you should limit for a variety of reasons. Some, which have been over-exposed in our diets (such as wheat), are likely to cause trouble if eaten in large quantities. Others should be limited because they easily become addictive, or because they can disturb your blood sugar balance.

There is a third category:

Class Three foods are those that should not be eaten at all except on Feast Days, because they are too destructive to the body.

CLASS ONE FOODS

Eat these foods freely on the Wright Diet.

Vegetables
You need a good variety of fresh vegetables, preferably eaten raw, and every day. Always choose unsprayed organically grown vegetables when you can get them. For

shops and farms near to you that sell them, see Useful Addresses on page 244. Or you can grow your own organic vegetables (see Useful Addresses for help with that too). But don't go without vegetables just because you can only get the sprayed variety, and don't *worry* about it if that is the case. Worry is much worse for you than a few chemicals – your daily vitamin C and your seaweed intake will protect you.

You can also sprout pulses, seeds and grains in your own kitchen, office or even hotel bedroom and create your own unsprayed vegetables (see the Sprouting Guide on page 190).

Lactic fermented vegetables such as Eden sauerkraut, beetroot, and mixed vegetables are rich in lactic bacteria just as yoghurt is. Eating them regularly as part of your salad will help to keep your intestines sweet and full of the healthy kind of bacteria. The onions are a very good substitute for pickled onions.

Grains
Whole grains such as oats, rye, barley, millet, maize (corn), rice and buckwheat may become an important part of your diet (depending on the outcome of the Food Tests – see page 112). Make sure that the grains you eat are unrefined, and the foods made from these grains too, such as pumpernickel bread, crispbreads and unsweetened biscuits. Wheat is not a Class One food. See the Class Two foods below to find out why.

Pulses
Dried peas and beans were staple foods for our peasant ancestors for thousands of years. They're exceptionally high in fibre and make an excellent alternative to meat. If your body likes them, make them a regular part of your

diet. Soya beans, haricot beans, chickpeas, butter beans
and so on are all pulses. As are lentils, mung beans,
alfalfa sprouts, aduki beans, and black-eyed beans too.
Many of these are best sprouted before cooking or eating
(see the Sprouting Guide, page 190) and some can be
eaten raw (see the recipes, page 187). Foods such as tofu
(a kind of cheese made from soya beans which you can
buy from health food shops), and humous made from
chickpeas, are also pulse foods.

Edible Seeds

Sesame, sunflower and pumpkin seeds, linseeds, and
melon seeds are all rich in oils that contain essential
nutrients for the body. Using them daily will enrich your
skin, help prevent a heart attack and reduce pain and
inflammation. But these oils are polyunsaturated and can
easily rancify, creating damaging chemicals called free
radicals that can be ageing and cancer promoting. So only
buy them fresh and unchipped and keep them in a cool
dark place. Some seeds, such as linseeds and sesame
seeds, are best ground in a coffee grinder before serving
to help digestion (or sesame seeds may actually come
through your body whole), but only grind what you need
for up to three days and keep what you don't use in the
fridge. Tahini (sesame seed spread) is an excellent food.
Sesame has one of the most stable oils. But don't roast or
fry any of the seeds. Cooking or browning any of these
sensitive oils will create free radicals. Linseeds are unique
in being the only vegetable source rich in an oil called
alpha-linolenic acid (otherwise found in fatty fish) which
helps to prevent blood clots and heart attacks. They are
also very soothing and healing to the digestive system
walls, and excellent for preventing constipation.

Seaweeds
Sea vegetables such as nori, wakame, hiziki and dulse are rich sources of iodine and trace minerals. You'll find them delicious. Buy them in health food and wholefood shops and use them in soups and casseroles regularly.

Fish
Fish is an excellent source of protein if your body likes it. The fatty fish (such as salmon, herring and mackerel) are higher in nutrients than white fish, and some of their oils help to prevent heart disease. Fish should be as fresh as possible. But it's all right to buy it fresh and then freeze it at home. Don't eat salted, smoked, tinned or commercially frozen fish because of the chemicals added. Smoked fish for instance is high in salt, and preserved with nitrates or nitrites which can cause cancer (and may also cause diabetes in the next generation). Shop-bought taramasalata (Greek cod's roe paté) contains artificial colour, but see the recipes for an original Greek colour-free version.

White Meat
White meats such as liver and kidney, chicken and turkey can be a good source of protein, especially if you can get them from a butcher who sells meat free of antibiotics and hormones (see Useful Addresses for details of a nationwide service). Don't eat meat that contains these additives more than once a week. Only eat beef liver if it is additive-free. Goose and duck are too high in fat for frequent use, but game (pheasant etc.) is higher in polyunsaturated oils and should also be additive-free. But look out for the lead shot.

Yoghurt
Cow's, goat's and sheep's yoghurt tends to be more digestible than milk because the milk sugar, lactose, which

causes many people difficulty, has been digested by the yoghurt culture. Go for plain yoghurt made from whole milk free from antibiotics and hormones, or make your own. Avoid 'creamed' or strained yoghurts as they're far too high in fat.

Cheese

Ideally the cheese you eat should be low fat and made only from milk from non additive-fed animals, and should be free of artificial colouring. It should most definitely not be processed or smoked. In practice only some goat's and sheep's cheeses, and a very few cow's cheeses fit these requirements (see the Organic Food Guide listed in Useful Addresses). Cottage cheese, Ricotta cheese (from Italian shops) and Feta cheese (from Greek shops and some delicatessens) come a close second. Feta (made from sheep's milk) is very salty. Soak it under water overnight and then change the water to remove salt (do not buy the Danish substitute for Feta cheese made from non additive-free cow's milk).

Vegetable Oils

The best oils to use are virgin olive oil and cold pressed sesame oil because these are the most stable, and least likely to rancify and cause free radical damage. They also have a long historical tradition – they've been used for many hundreds of years – whereas oils like sunflower, corn, safflower etc. have only been used for 50 years or so. It's best to get the nourishment of oils like sunflower oil from the seed itself, not from the oil which easily creates free radicals. If you do use these highly polyunsaturated oils, don't cook with them. Keep all oils in the cool and dark to avoid rancidity. Avoid the dark sesame oil – it is made from roasted seeds.

Fresh Fruit
Fruit is a good source of vitamins and minerals, and a
good way to keep up your alkalinity. Try to get unsprayed
organically grown fruit, and check when you come to the
Food Tests that fruit is what your body wants. Surprisingly
some of us do better without it.

Culinary Herbs
Use herbs freely in your food dishes but avoid herb salts.

Culinary Spices
Use spices too but only in their natural form e.g. cumin
and cayenne not barbecue sauce!

Vegetable Stocks and Cubes
These are very helpful for adding flavour providing
they're low in salt. Soy sauce and tamari (another form of
soy sauce) are extremely high in salt. Look out for
additives in stock cubes, especially lactose to which many
people are intolerant. See Savoury Concentrate recipe,
page 190, for how to get a salty flavour without eating
extra salt.

Fruit and Vegetable Juices
Freshly juiced or bottled juices are a good alternative to
coffee and tea. They're alkaline-forming too, and excellent on your Fast Day. Juices are strong – it's a good idea
to dilute them with springwater. Don't drink too much
orange juice. We're all getting over-exposed to it, and it's
becoming a common allergen (and frequent trigger of
headaches). Beware of aluminium lined packaging which
may leach into the juice and check labels for additive-free
juices. All purchased juices will have been pasteurised.

Herb Teas

Don't feel you have to drink herb teas to be healthy. Some taste awful, but lemon grass tea is particularly tasty if you can get it. Rooibosch tea (packaged in tea bags and available from health shops) tastes like Indian tea but is caffeine-free. Peppermint, lemon verbena and chamomile can be satisfying too.

Water

Tap water may contain toxic metals (lead, copper, aluminium), chlorine, agricultural and other undesirable chemicals. Get a Brita water filter (from delicatessens and health shops) or use springwater such as Evian, Volvic, Malvern etc. Perrier and the sparkling mineral waters are also excellent but slightly acidic so don't use them when you're trying to alkalise your blood (for instance when fasting).

CLASS TWO FOODS

You can eat these foods on the Wright Diet but in limited quantities. The maximum servings allowances do not mean you have to eat that much, or any at all!

Beef and Lamb

Use leaner cuts only and cut off any fat. You would do better to eat less red meat because of its fat content, but if you do eat red meat it's important to look for meat free of antibiotics and hormones. See Useful Addresses for sources.

Maximum Servings
Additive-free: 3 times a week. Non additive-free: once a week.

Wheat and Bread

Wheat is one of the foods we eat far too frequently in many forms. Not only has it become a common allergen, it is a common cause of constipation because of its gluten content (a very sticky protein), and can trigger slowed transit of food through the intestines (the cause of many problems). Limiting your wheat intake helps you to explore other grains such as oats, rye, buckwheat and millet (see recipes).

Maximum Servings

Wholewheat bread: 2 slices a day. Plus one other wholewheat serving (biscuits, pasta etc.) a day.

Milk

Cow's and goat's. Milk is a natural food for human and animal offspring until weaned. After that most species and many members of the human race lose the ability to digest milk properly. Exposure to milk and milk products is so frequent in our society that it is possible to have had a 'masked' reaction to milk since being weaned. Cow's milk also has a high fat content unless skimmed, but skimmed milk is usually only made from 'factory farmed' animals that are given antibiotics in their feed. A recent analysis of cow's milk also revealed 50 different pesticides. Drink only cow's or goat's milk from naturally fed animals, preferably whole, or not at all.

Maximum Servings

½ cup (¼ pint) daily.

Cheese

Most cheese contains considerable quantities of saturated fats and should be limited for this reason. Ideally the cheese you eat should be made only from milk from additive-free animals, and should be free of artificial colouring. It should most definitely not be processed or smoked. Check out your response to cheese on the Food Tests.

Maximum Servings
Cheeses outside the Class One category: ½ lb (225 g) per week.

Butter and Margarine

Most of us love butter but it's almost pure saturated fat. Choose unsalted varieties and be sensitive to the taste that can tell you when it's rancid. Avoid all hard margarines like the plague. They're as good as saturated too, and heavily processed. Even polyunsaturated margarines go through many chemical processes and have to be partially saturated. All margarines contain considerable quantities of distorted fatty acids about which there is growing concern among some scientists. If you choose to use a little polyunsaturated margarine check that it contains natural antioxidants such as vitamins A and E.

Maximum Servings
2 oz (50 g) of either per week.

Eggs

Eggs should be not only free range but from animals fed additive-free feeds. Check with your supplier. Although egg yolks are high in cholesterol this has not been shown to affect blood cholesterol significantly. You should check with the Food Tests that eggs are OK for you, however. Soft boil, bake or scramble. Don't fry.

Maximum Servings
3 eggs per week.

Nuts

Almonds, hazelnuts, walnuts, cashew nuts, chestnuts and brazil nuts are all good foods in reasonable quantities providing that they suit you. They are very concentrated foods however and should be limited unless you're using them as a meat substitute. All nuts should be unsalted and unroasted, whole and undamaged. They should only be chopped or ground just before use. Don't eat peanuts or peanut butter. They can carry a mould which is now recognised as carcinogenic, and peanut oil promotes atherosclerosis and artery disease. Desiccated coconut is very high in saturated fat.

Maximum Servings
½ lb (225 g) per week.

Dried Fruit

Dried fruit are highly concentrated foods and you can easily over-eat them. You avoid this if you soak them before you eat them. Choose only fruits which are free of sulphur dioxide (which makes them retain their natural bright colour) and mineral oil. Look also for organically grown dried fruit. Watch out for dried fruit that cause reactions (compulsive eating is a good sign).

Maximum Servings
¼ lb (115 g) a week.

Honey and Natural Sweeteners

Honey, maple syrup and date sugar are also very concentrated food sources – they can easily displace more of the bulky foods in our diets. Buy only the best sources and use them very sparingly as your grandmother would have done. Honey should not be 'produce of more than one country' or it will have been heated. Jams, fruit and carob spreads should be free of added sugar.

Maximum Servings
3 tsp of any one of these daily. ¼ (115 g) of any sugar-free spreads weekly.

Caffeine

Coffee, tea, chocolate and cola drinks all contain caffeine and related stimulants to which most of us have long been addicted. They can also cause breast cysts in women. Start to cut them down or out now.

Maximum Servings
Coffee from beans: 1 daily. Tea: 2 daily. Chocolate/cocoa: none. Instant coffee: none. Cola drinks: none.

Caffeine-free Drinks

Decaffeinated coffee, dandelion coffee and grain coffees (from health shops) are useful substitutes when you're cutting down on caffeine. But all coffee contains considerable roasted material (carcinogenic), so don't make them too much of a habit.

Maximum Servings
3 cups of any a day.

Alcohol

Alcohol is another very concentrated source of fuel and easily becomes addictive. Although a little alcohol seems to reduce some heart diseases, it is associated with many other diseases including cancer and strokes. Many forms of alcohol contain a lot of chemical additives. Look for organic wine and cider (see Useful Addresses page 244).

Maximum Servings
Daily: Wine: 1 glass. Real beer: ½ pint (300 ml). Organic cider: ½ pint (300 ml). Spirits: none.

CLASS THREE FOODS

These foods are *not* allowed on the Wright Diet.

Pork
In any form. Pork can transmit a parasite called trichinosis to humans when the meat is not cooked correctly. Almost all pork is infected with it. The trichinae hatch in the human body and burrow into muscles and tendons. The body forms capsules of calcium around the parasites which eventually cause pain whenever the infected person moves about. Autopsies show that 20 per cent of the population are infected.

Preserved Meats
Bacon, sausages and almost all tinned, frozen and preserved meats contain nitrites to keep them pink and prevent botulism. Nitrites cause cancer.

Salt
Don't add any form of salt to your food except ones that are balanced with, or higher in potassium. See Recipe section page 187 for how to get a salty flavour without eating extra salt.

Spirits
Whisky, brandy, etc. These are too concentrated for our blood sugar control to handle.

Smoked Foods
All smoked foods contain cancer-promoting smoke derivatives and very high salt, but most smoked foods now also contain yellow dye. If you can get smoked food that is genuinely prepared in the old-fashioned way, save it for your Feast Days.

Instant Coffee
Most instant coffee has added caffeine, and is definitely a highly processed food. Stick to old-fashioned beans.

Cream
Very high saturated fat. For Feast Days only.

Shop Frozen Food
Because of the additives. Home freezing is OK.

Lead Contact Foods
Tinned food comes in lead soldered tins (this is most tins at present although another process is said to be replacing it). Food grown or displayed near a busy road will also be high in lead.

Refined Flour Products
Bread, biscuits, pastry, doughnuts, sauces (except home-made). Also used as a filler in many processed foods.

Chemicals
Any foods containing artificial colours, flavours, preservatives or other chemical additives.

Fried Food

Frying promotes cancer-promoting and ageing factors in food. This includes the stir-fried method. Try to add oil to food only after cooking. Use polyunsaturated oils cold only.

Burned Foods

Burning and browning promotes cancer-promoting and ageing factors in food (see page 63). So don't burn the toast or drink high roasted coffees.

Recipes

The food you eat on the Wright Diet has a taste all of its own. Fresh and nourishing, but above all vital. And there's really very little involved in preparing any of our meals. Most of the meals we eat at Green Farm every day take no more than twenty or thirty minutes to prepare (one or two that I've included here do take a little longer). That time is nearly always spent in good company as one person chops a handsome salad and the other puts together some grains, fish, or pulses. When we have guests we all pile into the kitchen together and emerge half an hour later with a delicious banquet.

One of the nicest things about preparing these dishes is that they all smell good too. Because we don't fry, there's never the heavy odour of burned fat or oil in the house. Just the aroma of real foods served raw or cooked very simply.

Here are some of the utensils you will need:

Wooden chopping board
One or two sharp knives for salad
Garlic crusher
One or two thick-bottomed stainless steel pans
Brita Water Filter (from health shops)
Blender or food processor
Stainless steel pressure cooker
Freezer

You can do without the pressure cooker and the freezer, but they both help to make the Wright Diet a way of eating that you can easily incorporate into a busy lifestyle. I don't advocate using the pressure cooker for anything other than cooking pulses. If it's a matter of spending two hours hovering over a pan of beans, I know that I will very rarely do it, and nor I suspect will you. But chopping a salad and talking to friends for twenty minutes while the beans cook in the pressure cooker is a possibility and one that brings this tremendous potential for nourishment within our grasp. (Incidentally, we find that the pressure cooker reduces the flatulence potential of the beans almost completely!)

A freezer is marvellous for saving time too. I would never freeze my vegetables or fruit, but I do find it useful for other dishes. I double the quantities when I'm preparing pulse dishes for instance and put half away for later in the month. I also buy good quality fish when I see it and tuck that away in the freezer too. Of course it would be ideal only to eat foods that are fresh every day. But if I did I wouldn't also be running the Green Farm Nutrition Centre or writing this book!

Eating Out

Don't worry about eating out. We do it frequently. There's always something good on the menu (we usually have fish) and a talk to the waiter will usually persuade them to modify their cooking methods if need be. Of course you're not going to get that great big salad, and you're going to feel acidified by the end of the evening. Go home and eat some fruit to counterbalance the acidity (pineapple is great for this because it has enzymes that help digestion too). If you feel however that you've really overdone it, take some digestive enzyme tablets (available from good health shops for just this kind of occasion).

Acid/Alkaline Balance

All the main meals in the recipes are alkaline-forming because of the salads that you eat with them. Remember that the more salad you eat the higher the alkaline content of the meal will be. After a while you'll start to know when you feel a lack of alkalinity – you'll feel grumpy and uncomfortable. Your remedy is to make the next meal one that is high in alkaline-forming vegetables, or to take a mid-meal snack of fruit.

Some of the breakfasts – for instance eggs, toast, muesli or porridge – are acid-forming. To rebalance this you can either add alkaline fruits to your breakfast (dried figs, for instance, are one of the most alkaline foods of all), or make sure you have an alkaline snack mid-morning.

Good Food Combinations

All the meals given in the recipes follow the principles of good food combining unless otherwise stated. I find that some people are more sensitive to bad combinations than others. Following the Wright Diet will soon show you how you yourself can benefit from this principle.

Meat, Fish or Pulses?

A lot of the recipes I give for the Wright Diet are for pulses and vegetables. This is because I find that, on the whole, people know much less about how to cook these. I have given two or three meat and fish recipes and general guidelines for cooking both.

But the fact that the emphasis of the recipes is on vegetarian rather than animal protein is not meant to imply that you should eat one kind of protein in preference to the other. Only you can tell which way of eating is best for you.

Savoury Concentrate

Throughout the recipes I refer to 'savoury concentrate.'
By this I mean an equivalent amount of any concentrated
vegetable stock (either as a stock cube or a paste) PLUS
the appropriate amount of potassium salt to balance the
excess sodium, so that your food does not contain any
extra sodium.

For 1 teaspoon of savoury concentrate use

1 teaspoon Vecon
or 1 teaspoon Plantaforce
or 1 teaspoon Soy sauce
or 1 teaspoon Tamari
or 1 vegetable stock cube
(All available from health shops.)

PLUS

1 teaspoon potassium salt (Ruthmol and Trufree salt
replacer are two very good potassium salts available from
health shops.)

Sprouting Guide

Sprouts are full of nutrition. In the first few days the
vitamin content of these little seeds increases significantly. They're also excellent for keeping up your
blood sugar, a tasty addition to any salad.

Nothing could be easier than sprouting. In spite
of all the books and lengthy descriptions and expensive sprouting equipment around, sprouting comes
down to this:

You sprout seeds, beans and grains by soaking

continued overleaf

Sprouting Guide – *cont.*

them so that they start to germinate, and then keeping them warm and moist for a few days. They need to be rinsed a few times a day to keep them moist and to prevent the growth of moulds.

Soak them by washing them in clean water and picking out any obvious duds or bits of dirt. Then stand them to soak for the time given below (or overnight) in a jam jar. You can have one jam jar for each kind or you can grow them all together. When their soaking time is over throw away the water (some raw beans contain compounds that are undesirable until they have been sprouted).

It's easier to drain off the water without losing your sprouts if you put a little muslin over the top of the jam jar and hold it on with a rubber band. Then all you have to do is water them two or three times a day (more in hot weather or in a hot kitchen) and be ready to harvest your crop when it's ready. If you want your sprouts to go green (alfalfa, for instance), put them on the windowsill for at least a day or two. Otherwise it doesn't matter.

Seed	Soak	Rinse	Ready in
	hours	times a day	days
Aduki bean	8–12	3	3–5
Alfalfa	5–8	2–3	5–6
Chickpeas	8–15	3	3–4
Fenugreek	6–8	3	3–4
Lentils	8–12	3	2–3
Millet	5–8	3	3–4
Mung (bean sprouts)	8–12	4	5–6
Wheat (whole kernel)	8–15	2	2–3

BREAKFASTS

Breakfast really is the most important meal of the day. If you get breakfast right then staying on a healthy course for the rest of the day will be easy. If you try to go without it you'll probably come unstuck before lunchtime. Forget about breakfasts that come out of a packet – they're full of chemicals and sugar. Working your way through the recipes below should give you a whole new idea about breakfast. None of the meals suggested take more than five minutes, and all of them help keep your blood sugar supplied for several hours.

Porridge

We haven't found a better breakfast yet for giving you energy and keeping you satisfied for hour after hour – as the Scots always knew, of course. This version, just barely cooked, combines the nourishment of oats and millet to give you protein, iron, calcium, B vitamins and lots of bulk and fibre. (Oat fibre is superior to wheat because it's water soluble and much more digestible). You should be able to get organically grown porridge oats and millet flakes from a health shop. They must be porridge oats – ordinary oat flakes won't make good porridge.

Porridge oats 3 oz (75 g)
Millet flakes 3 oz (75 g)
Filtered water 1¼ pints (250 ml)
Freshly ground seeds (sunflower, sesame,
pumpkin and linseed) 1 – 2 tbsp

Put the oat and the millet flakes into a thick-bottomed pan together with approximately a quarter of the water. Mix to a smooth paste and heat gently over a low heat. Heat the rest of the water and mix it into the porridge, stirring gently for three to four minutes until smooth and ready to eat.

Serve with a good sprinkling of ground seeds and just a little honey, or with Banana Cream (see recipe on page 195), or with yoghurt, raw milk, or soya milk (which you can get from most health shops). Remember you can keep ground seeds in the fridge for up to three days but no longer.

This recipe makes 2 generous servings or 4 smaller ones. Preparation time 5 minutes.

Variations: You can make a delicious porridge by soaking chopped, dried fruit such as dates or figs overnight in a cup of cold water and then using the fruit and soaking water for making the porridge. If you don't have millet flakes simply use twice the quantity of oats.

To save bothering with weighing and measuring first thing in the morning use one cup of flakes to two cups of water (for one generous serving or two smallish ones).

Muesli

It's best to buy each ingredient separately and combine them yourself. That way you can be sure of the quality, although some health stores make good muesli bases to which you can add fresh or dried fruit. Try to get organically grown grains, and avoid packaged muesli that contains sugar and other additives. The recipe I give here is served with yoghurt as it's so much more digestible than milk.

Home-made muesli base of organic rolled oats, barley, rye and millet flakes 1–3 tbsp
Raisins or other dried fruit 1 tbsp
Apple or other fresh fruit 1
Plain yoghurt from additive-free milk 2½ oz (70 g)

Honey (optional) 1 tsp
Water 1 cup
Freshly ground seeds (as in porridge recipe)
1–2 tbsp

Soak the muesli base and dried fruit overnight in one cup of water (if possible), and stir in the yoghurt and grated apple just before serving it. Top with sprinkling of ground seeds, and honey if you need it.

1 serving.
Preparation time 2 minutes.

Variation: if you prefer not to use yoghurt, substitute apple juice, soya milk (from a health shop) or Banana Hazelnutshake (see opposite) instead.

Yoghurt and Banana

A Green Farm favourite. Next to porridge we find it the most satisfying.

Plain yoghurt from additive-free milk
(cow's, goat's or sheep's) 5 oz (140 g)
Banana 1
Freshly ground seeds (as in porridge recipe)
1–2 tbsp

Chop the banana into the yoghurt and top with seeds. Delicious!

1 serving.
Preparation time 2 minutes.

Banana Yogshake

One of the first dishes we concocted when we came to Green Farm. Perfect for children, as a snack, before a morning sports workout, or just for breakfast.

Plain yoghurt from additive-free milk
5 oz (140 g)
Banana

Blend in the liquidiser or food processor for 30 seconds.

1 serving.
Preparation time 2 minutes.

Variations: Banana Yogshake is even tastier with a dash of real vanilla essence.

Banana Hazelnutshake
A delicious dairy-free shake for a quick breakfast, mid-morning snack, or any time.

Hazelnuts 1 oz (25 g)
Filtered water ¼ pint (140 ml)
Banana 1
Honey 1 tsp
Fresh lemon juice 1 tsp

Grind the hazelnuts, and blend with the other ingredients in the liquidiser or food processor. If you want to remove the little bits of hazelnut skin, blend nuts and water together first and pass through a coffee strainer. Then reblend with other ingredients. For an even stiffer shake use less water.

1 serving.
Preparation time 2 minutes.

Banana Cream
This makes a deliciously creamy dressing for porridge, yoghurt or fruit dishes.

Banana 1
Water ⅛ pt (70 ml)
Blend in the liquidiser or food processor.

1–2 servings.
Preparation time 2 minutes.

Fruit Breakfast

Perfect for a hot summer's morning or a day when you're only eating lightly. Fruit as a breakfast will not last as long as a grain or yoghurt breakfast, so be sure you have a good mid-morning snack to keep your blood sugar sustained.

Any fresh fruit (some of our favourites are
melon, pineapple, grapes, mangos, pears
and kiwis) 4–8 oz (115–225 g)

1 serving.
Preparation time 2 minutes.

Variation: Soak 2 oz (50 g) of dried fruit (free of sulphur dioxide and mineral oil) and 2 oz (50 g) of nuts overnight in two cups of water and serve with a topping of freshly ground seeds.

Eggs for Breakfast

Lightly boil two eggs, preferably additive-free and free range: lower gently into cold water, heat to boiling point, boil for 5 seconds, then serve immediately. Turn out onto a warm plate and serve with a sprinkling of parsley and a little low sodium salt, or use egg cups. (Try to avoid eggs and toast together especially first thing in the morning. They're a protein-starch combination and likely to give you indigestion.)

1 serving.
Preparation time 5 minutes.

Toast
It's best to use grains other than wheat at breakfast. Most of them are more filling, and you need to lessen your dependence on bread. This also means you save your wheat allowance for later in the day. If you do make toast for breakfast try to get a good wholewheat loaf made from organic flour. There are now several sugar-free organic jams on the market, or try tahini and honey (using tahini, which is sesame seed butter, instead of butter). Try to get used to putting things straight on to bread without having to use butter or margarine.

Tahini and mashed banana make a good combination too (especially if you grill the toast, tahini and banana for 1 minute).

SALADS

Green Farm Salad
This is the salad we make and eat every day at Green Farm. It varies with whatever is available from the garden and who is in the kitchen! We go through phases of chopping finely, or leaving the vegetables in nice big chunky bites. Remember your salad should make up half to three quarters of everything you see on your plate. That's what gives you your daily alkaline input. So make a really big bowlful; it encourages everyone to have second helpings. When visitors come to stay they take very timid little portions. By the time they've been with us a week they're tucking into the salad as much as the rest of us. Serve it with any number of the side salads to vary the interest.

Choose from:
Green vegetables (cabbage, lettuce etc.),

Root vegetables (carrots, beetroot, celeriac),
Sprouted beans and seeds (alfalfa, bean sprouts, fenugreek seeds),
Celery, cucumber, mange-tout peas, onions, spring onion, string beans, courgettes,
Chinese cabbage.

Shred, grate, chop, slice as appropriate. Toss, dress and serve.

Variation: Add sunflower and pumpkin seeds.

Carrot and Beetroot Salad

One of my favourite salads. It tastes delicious and it's packed with beta-carotene (which the body makes into vitamin A) so it's marvellous for skin, and helps protect against ageing and cancer too.

> *Carrots 2 large or 4 small*
> *Beetroot 1 large or 2 small*
> *Celeriac (optional) ½ a large one*

Grate all the vegetables and toss together. Dress and serve as a side salad with a large raw vegetable salad and a starch or a protein dish.

2 servings.
Preparation time 5 minutes.

Green Lentil Salad

> *Sprouted green lentils 1 cup*
> *Onion 1 small*
> *Lettuce 4 leaves*

Slice the onion very finely, shred the lettuce and toss with the lentils and a simple oil and lemon dressing. Serve on a bed of lettuce wtih a large raw vegetable salad and a starch or a protein dish.

2 servings.
Preparation time 5 minutes.

Sauerkraut Salad

Sauerkraut is made from cabbage by a natural process of lactic fermentation just like yoghurt making. The method has been used and respected for centuries especially in Europe and Scandinavia where sauerkraut is considered very important for maintaining healthy digestion.

> *Sauerkraut (from health shop) 4 oz (115 g)*
> *Onion 1 small*
> *Cumin ½ tsp*
> *Juniper berries ½ tsp*

Shake out the sauerkraut, chop the onion finely and toss all the ingredients together with an oil and lemon dressing. Serve as a side salad with a large raw vegetable salad and a starch or protein dish.

2 servings.
Preparation time 5 minutes.

Vegetable Crudités

Snack on these any time, take them to the office, serve them as starters or as dips to go with humous or taramasalata instead of bread.

Carrots	*Cauliflower florets*
Celery sticks	*Cucumber*
Red, green and	*Celeriac*
yellow peppers	*Beetroot*
Radishes	*Courgettes*

The aim is to make stick shapes about 2 inches long or any shape firm enough to dip into something tasty.

Experiment with slices of carrot, beetroot, courgette, longways slices of cucumber and so on.

Prepare just before you need them and serve as a snack or an appetiser with humous, taramasalata, sesame paté or fresh goat's cheese.

As many servings as you chop, you'll never find crudités left over!

Tabbouli Salad

This makes a lovely summer salad, with a tang you'll really enjoy.

> *Bulgar wheat (from health shops) ½ lb (225 g)*
> *Tomatoes 4 oz (115 g)*
> *Cucumber ¼*
> *Medium onion 1*
> *Parsley 2 oz (50 g)*
> *Fresh mint 1 oz (25 g)*
> *or dried mint 2 tbsp*
> *Lemon juice 4 tbsp*
> *Virgin olive oil 4 tbsp*
> *Olives (optional – soaked to remove salt) 2 oz (50 g)*

Soak the bulgar wheat for 30 minutes in sufficient boiling water to expand the grains and make them edible. Chop the tomatoes and cucumber and slice the onion finely. Drain the wheat and rinse well in cold water. Toss all the ingredients together and chill slightly.

Serve along with a large raw vegetable salad and Plaki or Greek Bean Salad (wheat and beans make a whole protein), or stuffed into wholewheat pitta bread. Or take it to work for lunch and eat with raw vegetable crudités.

6 servings.
Preparation time 15 minutes. Ready to eat in 45–60 minutes.

Greek Bean Salad

A deliciously filling salad to serve with grain dishes and raw vegetable salads. You can make it in minutes if you have some ready cooked beans.

> *Haricot beans (soaked overnight or*
> *see quick method) 1 lb (450 g)*
> *Onions 3 large*
> *Parsley, chopped ½ cup (approx)*
> *Garlic 2 cloves*
> *Juice of 1–2 lemons*
> *Olive oil ¼ pint (140 g)*
> *Savoury concentrate ½ tsp*

Cover the beans with cold filtered water and simmer for two hours. Drain and allow to cool. Chop the onions, crush the garlic, and mix with all the ingredients.

4 servings.
Preparation time 8 hours soaking, 2 hours cooking, 5 minutes to prepare.

Quick method: Cover dried beans with boiling water in a pan, bring back to the boil and simmer for 5 minutes. Remove from the heat and allow to soak for 5 minutes, then cook under pressure in a stainless steel pressure cooker for 20 minutes. Cool and prepare as above.

4 servings.
Preparation time 35 minutes.

Oil and Lemon Dressing

There is really no more nourishing or pleasing dressing than this time-honoured favourite.

> *Virgin olive oil ½ cup*
> *Juice of 1 lemon*
> *Garlic 1–3 cloves*

Crush the garlic and pour the oil and lemon over it. Whisk gently with a fork and pour over the salad.

Sufficient for a salad for 2.

Herb Dressing

Add the following to the basic oil and lemon dressing – dried parsley 1 tsp, oregano 1 tsp, dill ½ tsp, cumin ½ tsp.

Sesame Dressing

Gradually add filtered water, a few drops at a time, to a tablespoon of sesame paté (see page 209) in the food processor, until you reach a smooth runny consistency.

LUNCHES AND LIGHT MEALS

Onion Soup

This soup will prove to you that you don't need to fry the onions. They taste just as delicious without. Adding the oil at the end of cooking keeps it fresh and digestible and gives you an even creamier taste, or you can leave it out altogether.

> *Onions 1 lb (450 g)*
> *Potatoes 1 lb (450 g)*
> *Stock made from 3 tsp of savoury*
> *concentrate 1½ pints (825 ml)*

Any finely chopped seaweed 1 oz (25 g)
Bay leaf 1
Wholewheat or buckwheat flour to
thicken 2 tbsp
Olive oil 2 tbsp

Chop the onions and potatoes and simmer in the stock for 20 minutes with the bay leaf. Divide into two, remove the bay leaf and blend until smooth. Take a little of the soup stock and make a paste with the flour in a basin. Gradually add more soup to the paste until it becomes quite liquid but without any lumps, then return it to the pan, stirring with a wooden spoon until the soup thickens. Do not boil. Remove from the heat, stir in the oil and serve.

2–4 servings.
Preparation time 30 minutes.

Variation: You may prefer to leave the soup unblended. Just take a little of the liquid to make the paste, then return the thickened stock to the pan stirring until it thickens.

Vegetable Soup

You can vary the contents of this soup depending on what's in season.

Tomatoes (soft) 1 lb (450 g)
Medium onion 1
Garlic 2 cloves
Medium potato 1
Stalks of celery 4
Medium leek 1
Courgette 1

Stock made from 4 tsp savoury
concentrate 2 pints
Bay leaf 1
Mixed herbs 1 tsp
Any finely chopped seaweed 1 oz (25 g)
Olive oil 3 tbsp

Pour boiling water over the tomatoes and peel off their skins. Chop the onion, crush the garlic, slice the potato, celery, leek and courgette. Simmer all vegetables, herbs and seaweed in the stock for about 20 minutes. Remove from the heat, take out the bay leaf, stir in the oil and serve. This soup is also good blended.

4–6 servings.
Preparation time 30 minutes.

Variation: Leave out the oil if you prefer.

Cauliflower Cheese

Crunchy steamed vegetables make a good substitute for rice or potatoes when you're eating a protein meal (see the Food Combining Chart, page 230).

Cauliflower ½ large or 1 small
Juice of 1 lemon
Savoury concentrate ⅓ tsp
Goat's cheese 3 oz (75 g)

Cut the cauliflower into quarters, steam for about 6 minutes (it should be crunchy but chewable). Work the lemon juice and the savoury concentrate into the goat's cheese with a fork. Serve over or with the cauliflower, together with a Green Farm Salad and side salads.

2 servings.
Preparation time 10 minutes.

Sesame Cauliflower

An even tastier version of cauliflower cheese, this time dairy-free.

Cauliflower ½ large or 1 small
Sesame paté 4 tbsp
Filtered water ⅛ pint (70 ml)

Steam the cauliflower as above. Blend the sesame paté with the water, adding more or less until you get the consistency you want. Serve over the cauliflower along with a Green Farm Salad and side salads.

2 servings.
Preparation time 10 minutes.

Baked Potato

I think everyone loves baked potatoes. They really take very little trouble and they let you know when they're ready by filling the house with a delicious smell. Potatoes are alkaline-forming so they add to your daily alkaline intake. They're also great for keeping your blood sugar going. Try not to use butter or margarine on your potato. There are so many more healthy alternatives – see the suggestions below.

Try to get organically grown potatoes (the skins of regular potatoes contain a fungicide many times above the safety limit). Wash one or two potatoes per person. Pierce each one shallowly with a fork (to let out the air). Bake in a moderate oven 375°F/190°C/Mark 5 for about 45 minutes.

Serve with humous, taramasalata, sesame paté, goat's cheese or simply with an oil and lemon dressing, along with a Green Farm Salad or a side salad.

Lamb's Liver

On the Wright Diet you should go for the simplest of
meat dishes. Grill or bake your lamb so that the fat drops
away and cut off all obvious pieces of it. Roast your
chicken in a brick or very simply in a baking tray. Always
try to buy additive-free meat (see Useful Addresses).

Liver is full of vitamins, particularly vitamin A and the B
vitamins. It's also a good source of iron, and a very
digestible meat. Only buy additive-free liver. An animal
raised on chemical feeds will concentrate those chemicals
in its liver.

> Onion 1 small
> Lamb's liver ½ lb (225 g)
> Bay leaf 1

Slice the onion and sweat in a very little water with the
bay leaf in a pan over a moderate heat. When the onions
are transparent put in the slices of liver and cook 3
minutes on each side. Serve with a Green Farm Salad and
side salads.

Baked Fish

Unless your body says no to fish I suggest you try to have
it at least once a week if not more often. Fish is an
excellent source of first class protein and rich in iodine
and other trace minerals that aren't always easy to find in
foods from the land.

If you don't have a good fishmonger near to you buy
fish when you do find something good and take it home
and freeze it. You can buy a whole box of Portuguese
sardines already individually frozen for very little money.
They'll keep you in sardines for weeks and to my mind
taste nicer than many fish four times their price. As they

come from the Atlantic they're less polluted too. It's good to get to know your fishmonger – he'll be willing to tell you where the fish come from and which are the freshest.

Don't buy anything from the Moray Firth; it's polluted with mercury.

Any fish – cod steak, plaice fillet, herring,
mackerel, etc. but not smoked – 1 small fish
or ¼ lb (115 g) per person
Garlic ½–1 clove
Fresh parsley (optional) A few sprigs

Ask your fishmonger to gut your fish and remove the heads. Then all you have to do is hold them under a firm jet of cold water to clean out the insides. Lay the fish in a baking tray or fish brick surrounded by ½ inch of water. Crush the garlic and put inside the fish or work into the skin. Bake until tender at 300°F/150°C/Mark 2 for about 20–30 minutes. Serve sprinkled with parsley, alongside a Green Farm Salad and a steamed vegetable if you wish.

Fish Curry
One of Brian's masterpieces. An excellent way to make fish palatable if you're not used to eating it.

Any white fish (cod, plaice etc.) 1½ lb (675 g)
Buckwheat or wholewheat flour 2 tbsp
Cold water 1 pint (600 ml)
Seaweed (flaked, crushed or powdered) 2 tbsp
Madras curry powder 3 heaped tsp
Fenugreek powder 1 heaped tsp
Cumin powder 1 level tsp
Savoury concentrate 2 tsp
Garlic 2 cloves
Onion 1 medium

Honey 1 tsp
Olive oil 3 tbsp

Skin the fish and cut into chunks. Make a paste with the
flour in a pan by adding a little of the water and stirring.
Work in the seaweed, curry powder, fenugreek, cumin,
and savoury concentrate gradually adding water as needed
to make a smooth sauce, heating slowly. Chop and add
the garlic and onion together with the honey and olive oil.
Then add the fish and continue to simmer very gently for
about 15 minutes.

Serve with a large raw vegetable salad and one steamed
vegetable (such as cauliflower, broccoli or mange-tout
peas).

4 servings.
Preparation time 30 minutes.

Taramasalata

A delicious whole protein snack or appetiser. The taramasalata that you can buy here or in Greece contains an
undesirable red dye. This recipe was given to us by Dr
Ribas of Athens.
Note: this recipe combines starch and protein.

Large potatoes 1½
Lemons 2
Medium onion 1
Cod's roe (not smoked) 10 oz (280 g)
Virgin olive oil 3 tbsp
Savoury concentrate ½ tsp
Garlic to taste
Sprinkle of parsley

Boil the potatoes, squeeze the lemons and chop the
onions. Skin the roe and remove any gristly bits. Blend

all the ingredients together adding water if necessary (the mixture tends to thicken later). Sprinkle with parsley. Taramasalata will keep for several days in the fridge, or you can make up a batch when cod's roe is in season and freeze it in meal-sized quantities.

Serve with raw sticks of celery, green pepper and carrot, or with hot wholewheat pitta bread. For a main course serve with a large raw vegetable salad.

10 servings.
Preparation time 20 minutes.

Sesame Paté

This was one of my more fortuitous discoveries when messing about in the kitchen. Sesame paté makes a delicious spread, or a tasty side serving for salad or baked potato, or a great alternative for cheese (see Sesame Cauliflower).

> *Juice of 1 lemon*
> *Tahini (sesame butter from health shops) 4 tbsp*
> *Garlic ½–1 clove*
> *Savoury concentrate ½ level tsp*
> *Curry powder (optional) pinch*

Squeeze the lemon into the tahini and stir in well until it forms a stiff paste. Work in the crushed garlic, savoury concentrate and curry powder. Use immediately or keep in the fridge (the flavour gets even better on standing).

2 generous servings.
Preparation time 5 minutes.

Sesame sauce: For a pouring sauce work a little water into sesame paté until you reach the consistency you want.

Pulse Dishes

A full serving of any of these dishes contains almost as much protein as you need in a day, more fibre than a 1 lb (450 g) loaf of wholemeal bread and no saturated fat. The high complex carbohydrate content will keep your blood sugar steady for many hours.

Falafels

These chickpea savoury balls are out of this world. They're delicious hot or cold, perfect for office lunches.

> *Chickpeas (soaked or sprouted, or see quick*
> *method) 8 oz (225 g)*
> *Onions 6 oz (160 g)*
> *Egg 1*
> *Cumin powder 1 tsp*
> *Coriander powder ¹/₂ tsp*
> *Savoury concentrate 2 rounded tsp*
> *Cayenne pepper pinch*
> *Fresh parsley ¹/₂ oz (15 g)*
> *or dried parsley 2 tsp*
> *Any chopped seaweed 1 oz (25 g)*
> *Olive oil for dressing ¹/₈ pint (70 ml)*

Preheat the oven to 325°F/190°C/Mark 5. Blend the chickpeas with all the ingredients except the olive oil and a quarter of the savoury concentrate, adding a little water if necessary (you may have to divide the ingredients into two lots for blending). Or use a mincer and combine chickpeas with the other ingredients by hand. Form into balls about ¾ inch in diameter. Line up on greaseproof paper in a baking tray and bake for about 30 minutes. Work half a level teaspoon of savoury concentrate into the olive oil, then toss falafels in oil before serving.

Serve with a large raw vegetable salad and Tabbouli Salad, or stuff into wholewheat pitta bread with salad.

6–8 servings.
Preparation time 1–3 days (for sprouting) plus 45 minutes.

Quick method: If you don't have sprouted or soaked chickpeas, cover the peas with boiling water in a pan, bring back to the boil, simmer for 5 minutes, allow to soak away from the heat for 5 minutes and then cook under pressure in a stainless steel pan for another 20 minutes. You should only need 10–15 minutes baking time after pressure cooking.

6–8 servings.
Preparation time 45 minutes.

Humous

Brian is the humous maker in our family. Every month or two he disappears into the kitchen. There's a flurry of creativity, the blender grumbles, garlic filters under the door, and finally a triumphant Brian and a bowl of humous emerges. There's nothing better. Good for heart and skin (sesame and garlic).

> *Sprouted chickpeas ½ lb (225 g)*
> *Sesame seeds ¼ lb (115 g)*
> *Garlic cloves 4*
> *Virgin olive oil or sesame oil 5 tbsp*
> *Juice of one lemon*
> *Savoury concentrate 1 tsp*
> *Water ½ (300 ml)*

Boil the sprouted chickpeas for half an hour. Grind the sesame seeds in a coffee grinder. Rinse the chickpeas in cold water. Blend all ingredients except the sesame seeds in a food processor with the water then add in the ground seeds (it's easier to make a purée of the chickpeas when they're more watery). Add more ground sesame to thicken if necessary.

Serve with raw vegetable sticks and/or hot wholewheat pitta bread as a snack or starter; or serve with a large raw vegetable salad and baked potato or briefly steamed cauliflower.

6 servings.
Preparation time 3 days plus 40 minutes.

Quick method 1: Sprouted chickpeas take at least three days. If you don't have sprouted peas simmer dried peas in water for 5 minutes, leave to soak for at least one hour, and cook for one hour (again simmering) before preparing as above.

Preparation time 3 hours.

Quick method 2: Cover the chickpeas with boiling water, simmer for 5 minutes, leave to soak for 5 minutes while you prepare the other ingredients. Throw away the water (the soak water from pulses should never be used as these foods contain anti-trypsin factors when raw), and cook in the pressure cooker for another 20 minutes. Then prepare as above.

Preparation time 40 minutes.

Plaki
This is a delicious and satisfying meal or side dish eaten regularly in Greek villages. I guarantee that if you like beans this dish will become one of your favourites. This dish is good served hot or cold.

*Dried haricot beans soaked overnight (or
see quick method below) 1 lb (450 g)
Tomatoes 1 lb (450 g)
Onion 1 medium
Fresh parsley a handful
or dried parsley 2 tbsp
Garlic cloves 2–3
Savoury concentrate 1/2 tsp
Chopped spring onions 6
Olive oil 1/4 pint (150 ml)*

Cover the beans with cold filtered water and bring to the boil. Chop the tomatoes, the onion and the parsley, and crush the garlic in a garlic crusher. Add tomatoes, onion, garlic, parsley and savoury concentrate. Cover and simmer gently for two hours. Remove from the heat when the beans are tender. Add the oil, sprinkle with more fresh parsley or chopped spring onion, and cool slightly, then serve with a large raw vegetable salad, wholemeal bread and wedges of lemon.

*2–4 servings.
Preparation time 2 hours.*

Quick method: Cover the dried beans with boiling water, simmer for 5 minutes, leave to soak for 5 minutes while you prepare the other ingredients. Throw away the water, cover with cold filtered water, add the tomatoes, onion, parsley, garlic and savoury concentrate and cook under pressure in the pressure cooker for 20 minutes. Add the oil and serve as above.

Preparation time 30 minutes.

Bean Feast
A really satisfying and creamy casserole dish that can be prepared in half an hour.

*Dried haricot beans (soaked overnight or
see quick method below) 1 lb (450 g)
Onions 1 lb (450 g)
Hiziki (or any dried seaweed) 1 oz (25 g)
Garlic cloves 2
Dried parsley 2 tsp
Savoury concentrate 2 level tsp
Curry powder (optional) 2 level tsp
Virgin olive oil 2 tbsp*

Put all the ingredients except the oil into a pan and simmer gently for 20 minutes. Remove from the heat, add the oil and serve. If you don't have ready-cooked beans use the quick method below.

Serve with a large vegetable salad. Adding bread or serving with rice will make this dish a complete protein.

4 servings.
Preparation time 8 hours soaking time plus 2 hours cooking.

Quick method: Cover the haricot beans in a pan of water and simmer for 5 minutes then allow to stand for 5 minutes while preparing other ingredients. Drain the beans and put all ingredients except the oil into the pressure cooker. Mix well. Cover the beans with boiling water, and cook under pressure for twenty minutes. Add the oil and serve.

4 servings.
Preparation time 30 minutes.

Variations: You can add ½ lb (225 g) of tomatoes, courgettes, green beans or any other vegetable to this dish. Simply check that there is enough liquid in the pan.

Lentil Nut Loaf
There isn't any short cut to this dish, but a nut loaf can be a delightful dish for Sunday lunch or for entertaining.

Whole lentils (green or brown) 5 oz (140 g)
Vegetable stock (made from 1 tsp savoury
concentrate) ¾ pint (450 ml)
Walnuts (or almonds, cashews or
hazelnuts) 6 oz (165 g)
Sesame seeds 1 oz (25 g)
Mixed nuts (freshly chopped) 2 oz (50 g)
Oat flakes 2 oz (50 g)
Onion 1 large or 2 small
Dried sage ¼ tsp
Thyme pinch
Cayenne or paprika pepper
(optional) pinch
Garlic 1–2 cloves
Any chopped seaweed 1 oz (25 g)

Bring the stock and the lentils to the boil and simmer gently until tender. Preheat the oven to 375°F/190°C/Mark 5. Blend the lentils to a smooth paste. Chop the onion, crush the garlic and sweat together in a pan in very little water over a low heat stirring constantly. Add the herbs and pepper and cook until soft (without using any unnecessary water). Remove from the heat and work in the lentils and all other ingredients. Line a loaf tin with greaseproof paper, turn the mixture into it, press down well and sprinkle with a few sesame seeds. Cover with a sheet of greaseproof paper and bake for 1½ hours, removing the greaseproof paper for the last 15 minutes. Cool in the tin.

Serve with a large raw vegetable salad and Onion Gravy or Tomato Sauce.

4–6 servings.
Preparation time 2¼ hours.

Tomato Sauce
This sauce makes a perfect gravy for the Lentil Nut Loaf,
Falafels etc.

> *Ripe tomatoes 1 lb (450 g)*
> *Onion 1 medium*
> *Wholemeal or buckwheat flour*
> *1 heaped tbsp*
> *Dried savory (herb) ¼ tsp*
> *Savoury concentrate 1 tsp*
> *Filtered water ½ pint (300 ml)*
> *Cayenne or paprika pepper*
> *(optional) pinch*
> *Garlic clove ½–1*
> *Juice of 1 lemon*
> *Ground ginger pinch*
> *Olive oil 1 oz (25 g)*
> *Kelp powder ¼ tsp*

Score the peel of the tomatoes, briefly pour boiling water
over them and remove the peel (throw away the water).
Chop the tomatoes and the onions and crush the garlic.
Simmer in a pan with the savory and the water. Add all
other ingredients except the flour, water and oil. When
cooked (5 minutes) blend. Mix the oil and the flour
together, gradually adding a little of the sauce until it
forms a smooth paste. Return to the pan and stir until the
sauce thickens. Serve while hot or keep in the fridge for
when you need it.

4–6 servings.
Preparation time 20 minutes.

Onion Gravy
A really simple gravy you can make in a few minutes.

Onion 1 medium
Vegetable stock (made from 2 tsp savoury
concentrate) 1 pint (600 ml)
Wholewheat flour 2 oz (50g)

Slice the onion finely and sweat it in a very little of the stock in a pan over a low heat. Then add the rest of the stock and simmer for 5 minutes. Now take a little of the stock and make a paste with the flour in a basin, gradually adding more of the stock to make a smooth gravy. Return to the pan and simmer while stirring until the mixture thickens.

Buckwheat and Vegetables
This is one of our favourite meals when the two of us are at home alone. Buckwheat is almost twice as high in protein as rice and we find it much lighter on the stomach and more digestible. It also takes next to no time to prepare.

Buckwheat grains (from any health shop) 5 oz (140 g)
Filtered water 1/2 pint (300 ml)
Savoury concentrate 1 tsp
Any vegetables, finely sliced
2 cups approximately

Wash the buckwheat in water allowing any cloudy water and bits of grit to pour away. Drain well. Put into a pan with the water and savoury concentrate (mixed in) and turn on a low heat. Cover and stir occasionally. After ten minutes put the vegetables on top of the buckwheat so that they can steam gently while the buckwheat is cooking. The buckwheat will be cooked when the water is completely absorbed. Toss and serve with a large raw vegetable salad and side salads.

2 servings.
Preparation time 20 minutes.

Variation: Use brown rice instead of the buckwheat and allow 35 minutes for cooking. Or use ⅔ brown rice and ⅓ green lentils to make a whole protein.

4 servings.
Preparation time 10 minutes.

DESSERTS AND BAKING

On regular days on the Wright Diet you don't have desserts or puddings. That's partly because they nearly always lead to undesirable food combinations, and partly because puddings with every meal are part of the late twentieth-century excess of eating.

If you want to serve something after a meal leave a decent interval (perhaps while someone does the washing up) and then put out a bowl of fruit.

Here however are some delicious cakes and puddings for when the occasion does arise. A slice of the bread or the fruit cake also makes an excellent mid-afternoon snack.

David's Low Fat Fruit Cake
This is a favourite among visitors to our courses when David, our Art Director, turns cook for the day.

> *Dried fruit (can be mixed raisins, chopped*
> *figs etc.) ½ lb (225 g)*
> *Honey 2 oz (50 g)*
> *Unsweetened fruit juice (pineapple,*
> *apple etc.) 6 tbsp*

Wholewheat flour (organic if possible) 6 oz (170 g)
Salt-free baking powder 2 tsp
Free range additive-free egg 1 large
Your favourite spice (nutmeg, allspice etc.
or mixed) ½ tsp

Preheat the oven to 325°F/170°C/Mark 3. Mix the dried fruit, honey and fruit juice in a bowl. Sieve the flour, baking powder and spices. Beat the egg and add it to the fruit mixture. Fold in the flour, mix with a wooden spoon and pour into a 1 lb (450 g) loaf tin lined with greaseproof paper. Cook for about 1 hour.

Variation: Make with two egg whites instead of one egg for a completely fat-free cake.

Banana Fruit Bread

A lovely moist fruit bread perfect for your mid-afternoon snack. This recipe makes two small loaves, which should last you the week if you bake them on Sunday.

Wholemeal flour (preferably organic) 1 lb (450 g)
Sultanas 2 oz (50 g)
Honey 2 oz (50 g)
Pear (must be ripe) 1
Bananas (the riper the better) 4
Cinnamon 1 tsp
Nutmeg 1 tsp
Rind of 1 lemon
Salt-free baking powder 4 tsp

Preheat the oven to 375°F/190°C/Mark 5. Blend the ripe pear and the bananas in the food processor. Sieve the flour and the baking powder. Mix the flour, sultanas, honey and spices in a basin. Add to the blended pear and bananas, add lemon rind and blend all ingredients until smooth. Divide between two 1 lb (450 g) loaf tins lined with greaseproof paper. Bake for about 35 minutes.

Oatcakes

These are perfect for spreading with sweet or savoury snacks. Cheese or humous for instance or a scoop of sugar-free jam. They're so easy to make, you might as well make a lot and keep them for the next week or two.

Oatmeal ½ lb (225 g)
Filtered water ¼ pint (140 ml)

Boil the water and stir it into the oatmeal. Knead for a few minutes. Roll out thinly with a rolling pin and cut into rounds with a cup or glass or pastry cutter. Bake for 30 minutes in a moderate oven 375°F/190°C/Mark 5.

Banana Ice Cream

This is a perfect dessert for entertaining on the Wright Diet.

Hazelnuts 4 oz (115 g)
Bananas 4 medium
Honey 2 tbsp
Molasses (optional) 1 tsp
Juice of 1 lemon

Grind the hazelnuts and blend all ingredients together. Put into the freezer for 2 hours. Reblend, divide into individual serving dishes or wine glasses and place in the fridge until required. Serve topped with a sprinkling of nuts or decorate with halves of grapes.

4–6 servings.
Preparation time 5 minutes. Freezing time 2 hours.

Mango Cream Dessert

Another perfect dessert for a special occasion.

Ripe mangoes 2
Bananas 4

Juice of fresh lemon
Cinnamon or other spice (optional) ¼ tsp

Peel mangoes and remove flesh with a knife. Blend with the bananas, lemon and spice. Pour into individual wine glasses and chill. Serve topped with chopped nuts or sliced fruit for decoration.

4–6 servings.
Preparation time 10 minutes. Chilling time ½ hour.

Carob Dates
Carob is an excellent alternative to chocolate, and it is caffeine-free too.

Almonds 12
Dates 12 whole
Sugar-free carob bar (from health shop) 2½ oz (75 g) bar

Blanch the almonds by pouring boiling water over them and lifting off the skins. Stone the dates and stuff them with the almonds, pressing them together again. Break the carob bar into small pieces and melt in a basin over a saucepan full of boiling water. When the carob is melted work in a little water until you get a smooth and thickish consistency. Dip the dates into the carob and lay them on waxed paper to cool. Serve in small paper cases.

DRINKS

Choose your drinks from the list of foods and drinks permitted. If you are eating plenty of raw vegetables and fruit and not eating any salt you may have little thirst. The theory that drinking lots of water is good for you is for people who flood their bloodstreams with junk food and chemicals. Drink when thirsty only.

Springwater, filtered water, fruit and vegetable juices. Grain coffees, herb teas.

Tea and coffee within your daily allowance: coffee (ground), 1 daily; tea, 2 daily; decaffeinated coffee, 3 daily.

Alcohol: daily maximum 1 glass of wine, or ½ pint of real beer or ½ pint organic cider (Aspall's). No spirits.

No chocolate drinks, instant coffee or cola drinks.

SNACKS

Take your snacks seriously on the Wright Diet. They're an important part of regaining your blood sugar balance and all that goes with it. Here are some suggestions.

Fresh fruit
Sunflower and pumpkin seeds
Banana yogshake
Banana hazelnutshake
David's Low Fat Fruit Cake (1 slice)
Banana Fruit Bread (1 slice)
Oatcakes served with
  Sesame paté
  Taramasalata
  Banana
Toast with any of the above
Banana Ice Cream
Falafels
Small bowl of muesli
Green Lentil Salad
Nuts

A Sample Week's Menu
On The Wright Diet

BREAKFAST		LUNCH		DINNER
1 Fruit	Snack*	Baked potato, Humous, Carrot & beetroot salad	Snack	Baked fish, Green Farm salad, Sauerkraut salad
2 Porridge	Snack	Greek Bean salad, Vegetable crudités	Snack	Liver & Onions, Green Farm salad
3 Banana hazelnutshake	Snack	Grilled sardines, Green Farm salad	Snack	Bean Feast casserole, Carrot & beetroot salad
4 FAST DAY Fruit	Fruit	Salad	Fruit	Baked potato, Green Farm salad
5 Yoghurt & banana	Snack	Tabbouli, Sauerkraut salad	Snack	Lamb cutlets, Green Farm salad
6 Muesli	Snack	Taramasalata, Vegetable crudités	Snack	Cauliflower Cheese, Green Farm salad
7 FEAST DAY Eat whatever you wish				

*Choose any snack from the list on page 222.

Acid/Alkaline Guide

The 'primitive' diet of our hunter-gatherer ancestors was, for hundreds of thousands of years, 65–75 per cent alkaline-forming and 25–35 per cent acid-forming[1]. Our own bodies function at optimum when the acid/alkaline balance of our foods is approximately the same.

Try to make 75 per cent of your diet alkaline-forming foods.

The acid/alkaline column refers to the degree of acid or alkaline effect of the food on the body (see Chapter 3), expressed in moles of alkalinity per 100 g of food.

ACID−/ALKALINE+

Alkaline Vegetables

Spinach	39.6	Horseradish	6.0
Beetroot	10.9	Tomatoes, raw	5.6
Potato, raw	10.3	Cabbage, raw	5.5
Potato, baked	9.4	Haricot, boiled	5.1
Carrots	9.4	Swedes, raw	5.0
Celeriac	8.7	Aubergine	4.5
Celery	8.6	Chicory	4.0
Mung beans, raw	8.4	Cucumber	3.1
Peas, dried	7.7	Mung beans, cooked	2.7
Lettuce	7.4	Lentils, raw	2.2
Parsnips	7.3	Peas, raw	1.3
Radishes	7.2	Lentils, cooked	0.6
Turnips	7.0	Onions	0.5
Watercress	6.9	Mushrooms	0.1

Acid Vegetables

Butter beans, boiled	−6.0	Asparagus, boiled	−1.7
Olives	−4.1	Broad beans, cooked	−1.6
Mustard & cress, raw	−2.3		

ACID−/ALKALINE+ − *cont.*

Acid Meats

Chicken liver	−28.0	Veal	−16.0
Calves' liver	−26.3	Turkey	−14.8
Lamb, lean meat	−19.2	Chicken	−14.3
Lamb's kidney	−17.3	Beef	−11.5

Acid Fish & Shellfish

Crab	−39.6	Salmon	−14.7
Lobster	−38.0	Oysters	−14.4
Prawns	−30.9	Cod	−14.3
Coley	−18.7	Halibut	−13.6
Lemon sole	−15.9	Haddock	−13.5
Trout	−15.5	Herring	−11.9
Plaice	−14.7	Mackerel	−10.9

Alkaline Fruits

Dried

Apricots, dried	41.7	Prunes	20.0
Figs, dried	35.7	Dates	12.2
Raisins	26.9	Peaches, dried	11.6
Currants	21.8	Figs, green	7.0
Sultanas	20.4		

Fresh

Rhubarb	12.9	Nectarine	6.3
Avocado	10.9	Orange	6.2
Lemons	8.6	Grapefruit	6.2
Blackberries	8.4	Raspberries	6.1
Apricots	8.3	Peaches	6.1
Banana	8.0	Honeydew Melon	6.0
Greengages	7.8	Grapes, white	6.0
Blackcurrants	7.8	Tangerines	5.4
Melon, Cantaloupe	7.5	Plums, Victoria	4.8
Loganberries	7.5	Gooseberries	3.8
Cherries	7.4	Strawberries	3.5
Grapes, black	7.3	Pears	3.4
Pineapple	7.0	Apples, eating	2.9

Acid Dairy

Edam cheese	−35.7	Cheddar	−6.3
Egg yolk	−33.9	Egg white	−4.9
Egg, whole	−16.7	Butter	−0.7
Stilton cheese	−7.9		

ACID−/ALKALINE+ – *cont.*

Alkaline Dairy

Skimmed milk	2.4	Whole milk	2.3

Acid Grains

Oatmeal	−13.9	Sago	−1.3
Wholemeal flour	−11.6	Tapioca	−1.3

Acid Nuts

Walnuts	−8.3	Hazelnuts	−3.9

Alkaline Nuts

Almonds	18.3	Brazil nuts	0.7
Chestnuts	11.3		

Miscellaneous

Honey	0.5	Honeycomb	−1.1

These figures were calculated for me by Richard Beale Ph.D.
The method used for these calculations is the one indicated in the original paper by Sherman and Sinclair, 'The balance of acid-forming and base-forming elements in food' (*J. Biol. Chem.* 3 (1907) 307–309).

Protein Guide

Your body needs somewhere between 30 and 70 grams of protein a day, depending on your body size, level of activity and state of health. Men generally need more than women because their bodies are larger. The amount you need also depends on how well your body utilises the protein that you give it. If your digestion feels good and you're using the Basic Supplement Programme your protein needs will be lower. If you do have digestive problems, on the other hand, you may need to take more protein and to be careful about your food combinations in order to get the same value.

All foods marked with an asterisk contain 'incomplete' proteins. That means they don't quite contain all the ingredients our bodies need to make them into human protein. When they're combined in the ways shown above, the two foods together form a whole protein. If you're eating meat, fish or dairy foods regularly you don't need to bother about this. They're all complete proteins. But if you want to eat some of your meals 'vegetarian' then it's as well to understand this simple principle. Often we combine the right foods instinctively. Beans on toast, for instance, or lentil soup served with a slice of wholemeal bread, are both whole protein meals.

FOOD	% or gm of protein per 100 gm of food		% or gm of protein per 100 gm of food

MEAT & POULTRY

Calves' liver	20.1	Lamb's liver, raw	20.0
Chicken	20.0	Turkey	23.2
Lamb chop, lean	27.8	Veal, raw	21.1
Lamb's kidney, raw	17.0		

FISH & SHELLFISH

Cod	21.0	Halibut	17.7
Cod's roe, raw	24.3	Herring, raw	16.8
Coley	23.3	Herring roe, raw	13.3
Crab	20.1	Lobster	22.1
Haddock, raw	16.8	Mackerel	19.0
Oysters, raw	10.8	Prawns	22.6
Plaice, raw	17.9	Lemon sole, raw	17.1
Salmon, raw	18.4	Trout	23.5
Sardines, raw	19.0	Tuna, canned	28.0

DAIRY & EGGS

Non-fat dried milk	35.9	Skimmed milk	3.6
Cottage cheese	25.0	Whole milk (cow's)	3.5
Hen's egg, whole	12.9	Yoghurt, low fat	3.4
Egg white	10.9	Goat's milk	3.2
Cream cheese	8.0		

GRAINS

Oats	14.2*	Buckwheat	11.7*
Wheat	14.0*	Millet	9.9*
Wheatgerm	26.6*	Corn (maize)	9.2*
Wheatbran	16.0*	Rice, brown	7.5*
Rye	12.1*		

Combine these with pulses for a whole protein

PULSES (BEANS, LENTILS, PEAS)

Soybeans	34.1*	Peas, dried	24.1*
Broad beans	25.1*	Black-eyed beans	22.8*
Lentils	24.7*	Chickpeas	20.5*
Haricot beans	22.5*	Lima beans	20.4*
Red kidney beans	22.5*	Tofu (soya cheese)	7.8*
Mung beans	24.2*		

Combine these with grains, seeds or nuts for a whole protein (except hazelnuts)

SEEDS AND NUTS

Pumpkin seeds	29.0*	Cashew nuts	17.2*
Sunflower seeds	24.0*	Walnuts	14.8*
Pistachios	19.3*	Brazil nuts	14.3*
Almonds	18.6*	Hazelnuts	12.6*
Sesame seeds	18.6*		

Combine these with pulses for a whole protein

	% or gm protein per 100 gm food		% or gm protein per 100 gm food
VEGETABLES			
Kale	6.0*	Mushrooms	2.7*
Brussel sprouts	4.9*	Cauliflower	2.7*
Broccoli	3.6*	Asparagus	2.5*
Parsley	3.6*	Watercress	2.2*
Spinach	3.2*	Potato	2.1*

These will add protein to whichever food group you eat

Food Combining Chart

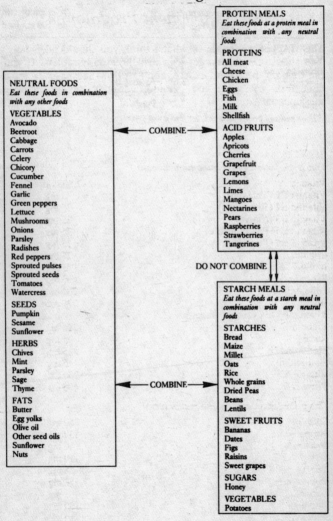

PROTEIN MEALS
Eat these foods at a protein meal in combination with any neutral foods

PROTEINS
All meat
Cheese
Chicken
Eggs
Fish
Milk
Shellfish

ACID FRUITS
Apples
Apricots
Cherries
Grapefruit
Grapes
Lemons
Limes
Mangoes
Nectarines
Pears
Raspberries
Strawberries
Tangerines

NEUTRAL FOODS
Eat these foods in combination with any other foods

VEGETABLES
Avocado
Beetroot
Cabbage
Carrots
Celery
Chicory
Cucumber
Fennel
Garlic
Green peppers
Lettuce
Mushrooms
Onions
Parsley
Radishes
Red peppers
Sprouted pulses
Sprouted seeds
Tomatoes
Watercress

SEEDS
Pumpkin
Sesame
Sunflower

HERBS
Chives
Mint
Parsley
Sage
Thyme

FATS
Butter
Egg yolks
Olive oil
Other seed oils
Sunflower
Nuts

← — COMBINE — →

DO NOT COMBINE

STARCH MEALS
Eat these foods at a starch meal in combination with any neutral foods

STARCHES
Bread
Maize
Millet
Oats
Rice
Whole grains
Dried Peas
Beans
Lentils

SWEET FRUITS
Bananas
Dates
Figs
Raisins
Sweet grapes

SUGARS
Honey

VEGETABLES
Potatoes

Basic Supplement Programme

This is a general guide to what I think you should take daily. You should be able to get it in just three daily tablets. If you can't match the values exactly don't worry. (See page 77 for a discussion of why you should consider taking regular supplements.)

Vitamin C Tablet

Vitamin C	1 gram

This is the formula of a good multivitamin:

Vitamin A	7,500 i.u.
Vitamin B1 (Thiamin)	75 mg
Vitamin B2 (Riboflavin)	75 mg
Vitamin B3 (Niacin)	75 mg
Vitamin B5 (Pantothenate)	75 mg
Vitamin B6 (Pyridoxine)	75 mg
Choline	75 mg
Inositol	75 mg
Paba	30 mg
Folic Acid	200 mcg
Biotin	75 mg
Vitamin B12 (Cyanocobalamin)	10 mcg
Vitamin C	250 mg
Rutin	25 mg
Bioflavonoids	25 mg
Hesperidin	5 mg
Vitamin E	200 i.u.
Vitamin D	400 i.u.

This is the formula of a good multimineral:

Calcium	250 mg
Magnesium	150 mg
Potassium	50 mg
Zinc	10 mg
Iron	8 mg
Manganese	8 mg
Copper	1 mg
Iodine	100 mcg
Selenium	10 mcg
Chromium	10 mcg
Plus Trace Minerals	

Food Analysis Table

	CAL	FAT	CARBO	FIBRE	VIT A	VIT C	VIT D	VIT E	VIT K	VIT B1	VIT B2	VIT B3 NIACIN	VIT B6
MEAT & POULTRY													
Calves Liver, raw	153	7.3	1.9	0	48700	18	10	.36	–	.21	3.1	12.4	.54
Chicken, light meat	116	3.2	0	0	tr	0	tr	.12	–	.1	.1	9.9	.53
meat & skin	230	18	0	0	tr	0	tr	–	–	.08	.14	6	.3
Lamb, chop, gr. lean	222	12.3	0	0	tr	0	tr	.15	–	.15	.3	7.2	.22
kidney, raw	90	3	0	0	330	7	–	.67	–	.49	1.8	8.3	.3
liver, raw	179	10	1.6	0	60400	10	.5	.69	–	.27	3.3	14.2	.42
Beef, lean, raw	123	4.6	0	0	tr	tr	tr	.15	–	.07	.24	–	.32
Turkey, light meat	103	1.1	0	0	tr	0	tr	tr	–	.08	.11	9.9	.59
Veal, fillet raw	109	2.7	0	0	tr	0	tr	–	–	.1	.25	7	.3
FISH & SHELLFISH													
Cod, raw	76	.7	0	0	tr	tr	tr	.66	–	.08	.07	1.7	.3
baked	96	1.2	0	0	tr	tr	tr	.88	–	.07	.07	1.7	.3
Coley, raw	73	.5	0	0	tr	tr	tr	.54	–	.1	.2	3.4	.4
steamed	99	.6	0	0	tr	tr	tr	.7	–	.12	.26	4	.6
Crab, boiled	127	5.2	0	0	tr	tr	tr	–	–	.1	.15	2.5	.3
Haddock, raw	73	.6	0	0	tr	tr	tr	–	–	.07	.1	4	.
Halibut	92	2.4	0	tr	0	tr	tr	134	–	.08	.1	5	.
Herring, raw	234	18.5	0	0	.150	tr	900	.31	–	tr	.18	4.1	.4
Lobster, boiled	119	3.4	0	0	tr	tr	tr	1.27	–	.08	.05	1.5	.
Mackerel, raw	223	16.3	0	0	150	tr	700	–	–	.09	.35	8	.
Oysters, raw	51	.9	tr	0	250	tr	tr	99	–	.1	.2	1.5	.0
Plaice, raw	91	2.2	0	0	tr	tr	tr	–	–	.3	.1	3.2	.4
Roe, cod, raw	113	1.7	0	0	466	30	80	9.54	–	1.5	1	1.5	.3
Roe, herring, raw	80	3	0	0	–	5	–	–	–	.2	.5	2	.
Salmon, Atlantic, raw	182	12	0	0	tr	tr	tr	–	–	.2	.15	7	.7
canned	155	8.2	0	0	299	tr	42	2.24	–	.04	.18	7	.4
Sardines, Pacific, raw	157	9	0	0	–	–	1150	1170	–	–	–	–	.2
Prawns, boiled	107	1.8	0	0	tr	tr	tr	–	–	–	–	–	.
Lemon Sole, raw	81	1.4	0	0	tr	tr	tr	–	–	.09	.08	3.5	.
Trout, brown, steamed	135	4.5	0	0	tr	tr	–	–	–	–	–	–	.
Tuna, canned in water	119	.8	0	0	–	–	–	–	–	–	.1	13	.

FOLIC ACID	VIT B12	VIT B5	BIOTIN	CA*	P	MG	K	NA	FE	CU	MN	ZN	SE	CR	S	CL
240	100	8.4	39	7	360	20	330	93	8	11	.17	7.8	43	.06	240	89
12	tr	1.2	2	10	210	27	330	72	.5	.14	.02	.7	12	.03	210	70
8	tr	.9	2	10	160	20	260	70	.7	.16	-	1	-	-	-	69
4	2	.7	2	9	240	28	380	75	2.1	.19	.02	4.1	18	.03	270	90
31	55	4.3	37	10	260	17	270	220	7.4	.42	-	2.4	-	-	180	270
220	84	8.2	41	7	370	19	290	76	9.4	8.7	-	3.9	-	-	230	83
10	2	1.3	tr	7	180	20	350	61	2.1	.14	-	4.3	-	-	190	59
8	1	.8	1	6	200	25	320	43	.5	.11	.02	1.2	-	.03	210	42
5	1	.6	tr	8	260	25	360	110	1.2	-	.02	3	-	.03	220	68
12	2	.2	3	16	170	23	320	77	.3	.06	-	.4	-	-	-	110
12	2	.2	3	22	190	26	350	340	.4	.07	-	.5	43	-	230	520
-	4	.38	7	14	190	23	260	73	.5	-	-	-	-	-	190	200
-	5	.4	8	19	250	31	350	97	.6	-	-	-	-	-	270	83
20	tr	.6	tr	29	350	48	270	370	1.3	4.8	.02	5.5	-	.03	470	570
13	1	.2	5	18	170	23	300	120	.6	.19	-	.3	-	-	220	160
12	1	.3	5	10	190	17	260	84	.5	.05	-	-	-	-	190	60
5	6	1	10	33	210	29	340	67	.8	.12	-	.5	-	-	190	76
17	1	1.63	5	62	280	34	260	330	.8	1.7	-	1.8	63	-	510	530
-	10	1	7	24	240	30	360	130	1	.19	-	.5	-	-	180	97
-	15	.5	10	190	270	42	260	510	6	7.6	-	45	65	-	250	820
10	2	.8	-	51	180	22	280	120	.3	.05	-	.5	-	-	240	170
-	10	3	13	-	-	-	-	-	-	-	-	-	-	-	-	-
-	5	.49		-	-	-	-	-	-	-	-	-	-	-	-	-
26	5	2	5	27	280	26	310	98	.7	.2	-	.8	-	-	170	59
12	4	.5	5	93	240	30	300	570	1.4	.09	-	.9	-	-	220	880
16	17	1	24	33	215	24	-	-	1.8	-	-	-	-	-	-	-
-	-	-	-	150	350	42	260	1590	1.1	.7	-	1.6	-	-	370	2550
11	1	.3	5	17	200	17	230	95	.5	.1	-	-	-	-	200	97
-	-	-	-	36	270	31	370	88	1	-	-	-	-	-	220	70
15	2.2	.3	3	16	200	-	280	40	1.6	.01	.02	.04	-	.03	-	-

For key to chemicals see page 243.

	CAL	FAT	CARBO	FIBRE	VIT A	VIT C	VIT D	VIT E	VIT K	VIT B1	VIT B2	VIT B3 NIACIN	VIT B6
FRUIT													
Apples, eating	46	tr	11.9	2	50	3	0	.2	-	.04	.02	.1	.03
Apricots	28	tr	6.7	2.1	2505	7	0	-	-	.04	.05	.6	.07
Apricots, dried	182	tr	43.4	24	6000	tr	0	-	-	tr	.2	3	.17
Avocado	223	22.2	1.8	2	167	15	-	4.77	-	.1	.1	1	.42
Banana	79	.3	19.2	3.4	334	10	0	.3	-	.04	.07	.6	.51
Blackcurrants	28	tr	6.6	8.7	334	200	0	1.49	-	.03	.06	.3	.08
Currants	243	tr	63.1	6.5	50	0	0	-	-	.03	.08	.5	.3
Cherries	47	tr	11.9	1.7	200	5	0	.15	-	.05	.07	.3	.05
Blackberries	29	tr	6.4	7.3	167	20	0	5.22	-	.03	.04	.4	.05
Dates	248	tr	63.9	8.7	83	0	0	-	-	.07	.04	2	.15
Figs, green	41	tr	9.5	2.5	835	2	0	-	-	.06	.05	.4	.1
Figs, dried	213	tr	52.9	18.5	83	0	0	-	-	.1	.08	1.7	.18
Gooseberries	37	tr	9.2	3.5	300	40	0	.6	-	.04	.03	.3	.02
Grapefruit	22	tr	5.3	.6	tr	40	0	.45	-	.05	.02	.2	.03
Grapes, black	61	tr	15.5	.4	tr	4	0	-	-	.04	.02	.3	
Grapes, white	63	tr	16.1	.9	tr	4	0	-	-	.04	.02	.3	
Greengages	47	tr	11.8	2.6	-	3	0	1.04	-	.05	.03	.4	.0
Lemons	15	tr	3.2	5.2	tr	80	0	-	-	.05	.04	.2	.1
Loganberries	17	tr	3.4	6.2	133	35	0	.3	-	.02	.03	.4	.0
Mangoes	59	tr	15.3	1.5	2000	30	0	-	-	.03	.04	.3	
Melon, Canteloupe	24	tr	5.3	1	3340	25	0	.15	-	.05	.03	.5	.0
Honeydew	21	tr	5	.9	167	25	0	.15	-	.05	.03	.5	.0
Watermelon	21	tr	5.3	-	33	5	0	.15	-	.02	.02	.2	.0
Nectarine	50	tr	12.4	2.4	835	8	0	-	-	.02	.05	1	.0
Orange	35	tr	8.5	2	83	50	0	.3	-	.1	.03	.2	.0
Peaches	37	tr	9.1	1.4	835	8	0	-	-	.02	.05	1	.0
Peaches, dried	212	tr	53	14.3	3340	tr	0	-	-	tr	.19	5.3	
Pears	41	tr	10.6	2.3	16.7	3	0	tr	-	.03	.03	.2	.1
Pineapple	46	tr	11.6	1.2	100	25	0	-	-	.08	.02	.2	
Plums, Victoria	38	tr	9.6	2.1	367	3	0	1.04	-	.05	.03	.5	
Prunes	161	tr	40.3	16.1	1670	tr	0	-	-	.1	.2	1.5	
Raspberries	25	tr	5.6	7.4	134	25	0	.45	-	.02	.03	.4	
Raisins	246	tr	64.4	6.8	50	0	0	-	-	.1	.08	.5	
Rhubarb	6	tr	1	2.6	100	10	0	.3	-	.01	.03	.3	
Strawberries	26	tr	6.2	2.2	50	60	0	.3	-	.02	.03	.4	
Sultanas	250	tr	64.7	7	50	0	0	1.04	-	.1	.08	.5	
Tangerines	34	tr	8	1.9	167	30	0	-	-	.07	.02	.2	

FOLIC ACID	VIT B12	VIT B5	BIOTIN	CA	P	MG	K	NA	FE	CU	MN	ZN	SE	CR	S	CL
5	0	.1	.3	4	8	5	120	2	.3	.04	.035	.1	.45	.015	6	1
5	0	.3	-	17	21	12	320	tr	.4	.12	.01	.1	-	.015	6	tr
14	0	.7	-	92	120	65	1880	56	4.1	.27	-	.2	-	-	160	35
66	0	1.07	3.2	15	31	29	400	2	1.5	.21	-	-	-	-	19	6
22	0	.26	-	7	28	42	350	1	.4	.16	.13	.2	.95	.015	13	79
-	0	.4	2.4	60	43	17	370	3	1.3	.14	-	-	-	-	33	48
11	0	.1	-	95	40	36	710	20	1.8	.48	-	.1	-	-	31	16
8	0	.26	.4	16	17	10	280	3	.4	.07	-	.1	-	-	7	tr
-	0	.25	.4	63	24	30	210	4	.9	.12	-	-	-	-	9	22
21	0	.8	-	68	64	59	780	5	1.6	.21	-	.3	-	-	51	290
-	0	.3	-	34	32	20	270	2	.4	.06	-	.3	-	-	13	18
9	0	.44	-	280	92	92	1010	87	4.2	.24	-	.9	-	-	81	170
-	0	.3	.1	19	19	9	170	1	.6	.15	-	.1	-	-	14	7
12	0	.28	1	17	16	10	230	1	.3	.06	.01	.1	-	.015	5	1
6	0	.05	.3	4	16	4	320	2	.3	.08	-	.1	-	-	7	tr
6	0	.05	.3	19	22	7	250	2	.3	.1	.065	.1	-	.015	9	tr
3	0	.2	tr	17	23	8	310	1	.4	.08	-	.1	-	-	3	1
-	0	.23	.5	110	21	12	160	6	.4	.26	-	.1	-	-	12	5
-	0	.24	-	35	24	25	260	3	1.4	.14	-	-	-	-	18	16
-	0	.16	-	10	13	18	190	7	.5	.12	-	-	-	-	-	-
0	0	.23	-	19	30	20	320	14	.8	.04	.01	.1	-	.015	12	44
0	0	.23	-	14	9	13	220	20	.2	.04	-	.1	-	-	6	45
3	0	1.55	-	5	8	11	120	4	.3	.03	.026	.1	-	.015	-	-
5	0	.15	-	4	24	13	270	9	.5	.06	-	.1	-	-	10	5
7	0	.25	1	41	24	13	200	3	.3	.07	.008	.2	1.3	.012	9	3
3	0	.15	.2	5	19	8	260	3	.4	.05	.01	.1	.4	.015	6	tr
4	0	.3	-	36	120	54	1100	6	6.8	.63	-	-	-	-	240	11
4	0	.07	.1	8	10	7	130	2	.2	.15	.01	.1	.6	.015	5	tr
4	0	.16	tr	12	8	17	250	2	.4	.08	1.2	.1	.55	.015	3	29
3	0	.15	tr	11	16	7	190	2	.4	.1	-	tr	-	-	4	tr
4	0	.46	tr	38	83	27	860	12	2.9	.16	-	-	-	-	19	3
-	0	.24	1.9	41	29	22	220	3	1.2	.21	-	-	-	-	17	22
4	0	.1	-	61	33	42	860	52	1.6	.24	-	.1	-	-	23	9
4	0	.08	-	100	21	14	430	2	.4	.13	-	-	-	-	8	87
0	0	.34	1.1	22	23	12	160	2	.7	.13	-	.1	-	-	13	18
-	0	.1	-	52	95	35	860	53	1.8	.35	-	.1	-	-	44	16
-	0	.2	-	42	17	11	160	2	.3	.09	-	.1	-	-	10	2

	CAL	FAT	CARBO	FIBRE	VIT A	VIT C	VIT D	VIT E	VIT K	VIT B1	VIT B2	VIT B3 NIACIN	VIT B6
VEGETABLES													
Asparagus, boiled	18	tr	1.1	1.5	835	20	0	3.7	60	.1	.08	.8	.04
Broad beans, boiled	48	.6	7.1	4.2	417	15	0	tr	–	.1	.04	3	–
Butter beans, boiled	95	.3	17.1	5.1	tr	0	0	–	–	–	–	–	–
Butter beans, raw	273	1.1	49.8	21.6	tr	0	0	–	–	.45	.13	2.5	.58
Chickpeas	373	5	61	5	50	–	0	–	–	.31	.15	2	.5
Green beans	37	.2	7	1	600	20	0	–	14	.08	.11	.5	.08
Haricot beans, boiled	93	.5	16.6	7.4	tr	0	0	–	–	–	–	–	–
Haricot beans, raw	271	1.6	45.5	25.4	tr	0	0	–	–	.45	.13	2.5	.56
Lima beans	126	.5	22	1.8	290	30	0	–	–	.24	.12	1.4	.6
Mung beans, cooked	106	4.2	11.4	6.4	273	tr	2.4	–	–	.09	.04	.4	.09
Mung beans, raw	231	1	35.6	22	40	tr	0	–	–	.45	.2	2	.3
Mung beans, sprouted	–	.2	6.6	–	20	20	–	–	–	.14	.14	.8	–
Red Kidney beans, raw	272	1.7	45	25	tr	tr	0	–	–	.54	.18	2	.4
Runner beans, raw	26	.2	3.9	2.9	668	20	0	.3	–	.05	.1	.9	.07
Soybean Curd, tofu	79	4.2	2.4	.1	0	0	0	–	–	.06	.03	.1	–
Soybeans	434	18	34	5	80	–	0	–	–	1.1	.3	2.2	.5
Aubergine	14	tr	3.1	2.5	tr	5	0	–	–	.05	.03	.8	.0
Beet greens	23	.3	5	1.3	6100	30	0	–	–	.1	.22	.4	
Beetroot, raw	28	tr	6	3.1	tr	6	0	0	–	.03	.05	.1	.0
Broccoli tops, raw	23	tr	2.5	3.6	4175	110	0	1.94	–	.1	.3	1	.2
Brussels Sprouts	26	tr	2.7	4.2	668	90	0	1.49	–	.1	.15	.7	.2
Cabbage, red, raw	20	tr	3.5	3.4	33	55	0	.3	125	.06	.05	.3	.2
Cabbage, savoy, raw	26	tr	3.3	3.1	501	60	0	.3	–	.06	.05	.3	.1
Cabbage, white, raw	22	tr	3.8	2.7	tr	40	0	.3	–	.06	.05	.3	.1
Cabbage, winter, raw	22	tr	2.8	3.4	501	55	0	.3	–	.06	.05	.3	.1
Carrots, old, raw	23	tr	5.4	2.9	20000	6	0	.75	–	.06	.05	.6	.1
Cauliflower, raw	13	tr	1.5	2.1	50	60	0	.3	–	.1	.1	.6	
Celeriac, boiled	14	tr	2	4.9	0	4	0	–	–	.04	.04	.5	
Celery, raw	8	tr	1.3	1.8	tr	7	0	.3	–	.03	.03	.3	
Chicory, raw	9	tr	1.5	–	tr	4	0	–	–	.05	.05	.5	.0
Cucumber	10	.1	1.8	.4	tr	8	0	tr	–	.04	.04	.2	.0
Garlic	100	tr	30	–	tr	15	–	–	–	.5	tr	.5	
Horseradish, raw	59	tr	11	8.3	0	120	0	–	–	.05	.03	.5	
Laverbread	52	3.7	1.6	3.1	–	5	0	1.64	–	.03	.1	.6	
Leeks, raw	31	tr	6	3.1	66.8	18	0	1.19	–	.1	.05	.6	
Lentils, cooked	99	.5	17	3.7	33	tr	0	–	–	.11	.04	.4	
Lentils, raw	304	1	53.2	11.7	100	tr	0	–	–	.5	.2	2	

FOLIC ACID	VIT B12	VIT B5	BIOTIN	CA	P	MG	K	NA	FE	CU	MN	ZN	SE	CR	S	CL
30	0	.13	.4	26	85	10	240	2	.9	.2	.18	.3	-	-	47	
-	0	3.8	2.1	21	99	28	230	20	1	.43	-	-	-	-	27	
-	0	-	-	19	87	33	400	16	1.7	.16	-	1	-	-	47	
110	0	1	-	85	320	164	1700	62	5.9	1.22	-	2.8	-	-	110	
200	0	1.3	10	150	330	-	800	26	7	-	-	-	-	-	-	
44	0	.2	-	56	44	30	240	7	.8	.04	.27	.3	.6	.06	-	
0	-	-	-	65	120	45	320	15	2.5	.14	-	1	-	-	46	
-	0	.7	-	180	310	180	1160	43	6.7	.61	-	2.8	-	-	170	
110	0	1	-	50	142	180	650	2	2.8	.18	.54	.8	-	.06	-	
20	0	-	-	34	100	51	270	820	2.6	.29	-	-	-	-	61	
140	0	-	-	100	330	170	850	28	8	.97	-	-	-	-	190	
-	-	-	-	20	64	-	224	5	1.3	-	-	-	-	-	-	
130	0	.5	-	140	410	180	1160	40	6.7	.61	-	2.8	-	-	170	
60	0	.05	.7	27	47	27	280	2	.8	.07	-	.4	-	-	-	
-	0	-	-	130	130	110	40	7	2	-	-	-	-	-	-	
170	0	1.7	60	230	550	265	1700	5	8	-	-	-	-	-	-	
20	0	.22	-	10	12	10	240	3	.4	.08	-	-	-	-	9	
-	0	.25	2.7	120	40	-	570	130	3.3	-	-	-	-	-	-	
90	0	.12	tr	25	32	15	300	84	.4	.07	.08	.4	-	.03	-	
130	0	1	.5	100	67	18	340	12	1.5	.07	.056	.6	-	.03	-	
110	0	.4	.4	32	65	19	380	4	.7	.06	-	.5	-	-	-	
90	0	.32	.1	53	32	17	300	32	.6	.09	.06	.3	2.3	.03	68	
90	0	.21	.1	75	68	20	260	23	.9	.07	-	.3	-	-	88	
26	0	.21	.1	44	36	13	280	7	.4	.03	-	.3	-	-	-	
90	0	.21	.1	57	54	17	390	7	.6	.06	-	.4	-	-	-	
15	0	.25	.6	48	21	12	220	95	.6	.08	-	.04	-	-	7	
39	0	.6	1.5	21	45	14	350	8	.5	.03	-	.3	.65	.03	-	
-	0	-	-	47	71	12	400	28	.8	.13	-	-	-	-	13	
12	0	.4	.1	52	32	10	280	140	.6	.11	-	.1	-	-	15	
52	0	-	-	18	21	13	180	7	.7	.14	-	.2	-	-	13	
16	0	.3	.4	23	24	9	140	13	.3	.09	-	.1	-	-	11	
-	-	-	-	30	200	-	550	20	1.5	tr	-	-	-	-	-	
-	0	-	-	120	70	36	580	8	2	.14	-	-	-	-	210	
47	0	-	-	20	51	31	220	560	3.5	.12	-	.8	-	-	-	
-	0	.12	1.4	63	43	10	310	9	1.1	.1	-	.1	-	-	-	
5	0	.31	-	13	77	25	210	12	2.4	.19	-	1	-	-	39	
35	0	1.36	-	39	240	77	670	36	7.6	.58	-	3.1	-	-	120	

	CAL	FAT	CARBO	FIBRE	VIT A	VIT C	VIT D	VIT E	VIT K	VIT B1	VIT B2	VIT B3 NIACIN	VIT B6
VEGETABLES—*cont.*													
Lettuce	12	.4	1.2	1.5	1670	15	0	.75	–	.07	.08	.3	.07
Marrow, raw	16	tr	3.7	1.8	50	5	0	tr	–	tr	tr	.3	.06
Mushrooms	13	.6	0	2.5	0	3	0	tr	–	.1	.4	4	.1
Mustard & Cress, raw	10	tr	.9	3.7	835	40	0	1.04	–	–	–	–	–
Olives	103	11	tr	4.4	300	0	0	–	–	tr	tr	tr	.02
Onions	23	tr	5.2	1.3	0	10	0	tr	–	.03	.05	.2	.1
Parsley, raw	21	tr	tr	9.1	11690	150	0	2.68	–	.15	.3	1	.2
Parsnips, raw	49	tr	11.3	4	tr	15	0	1.49	–	.1	.08	1	.1
Peas, raw	67	.4	10.6	5.2	501	25	0	tr	–	.32	.15	2.5	.16
Peas, split, dried, raw	310	1	56.6	11.9	250	tr	0	tr	–	.7	.2	3.2	.13
Peppers, Green	15	.4	2.2	.9	334	100	0	1.19	–	tr	.03	.7	.17
Potato, baked	85	.1	20.3	2	tr	10	0	.15	–	.08	.03	1	.14
Potato, old, raw	87	.1	20.8	2.1	tr	20	0	.15	3	.11	.04	1.2	.25
Radishes, raw	15	tr	2.8	1	tr	25	0	0	–	.04	.02	.2	.1
Spinach	30	.5	1.4	6.3	10000	25	0	2.98	–	.07	.15	.4	.18
Swedes, raw	21	tr	4.3	2.7	tr	25	0	0	–	.06	.04	1.2	.2
Sweet Potato	91	.6	21.5	2.5	6680	25	0	4	–	.1	.06	.8	.22
Sweetcorn, canned	76	.5	16.1	5.7	350	5	0	.75	–	.05	.08	1.2	.16
Sweetcorn, raw	127	2.4	23.7	3.7	400	12	0	1.19	–	.15	.08	1.8	.19
Swiss Chard, steamed	18	.2	3.33	–	5400	16	–	–	–	.04	.11	.4	
Tomatoes, raw	14	tr	2.8	1.5	1002	20	0	1.79	–	.06	.04	.7	.1
Turnip Greens	35	.3	5	.8	7600	139	0	–	650	.2	.4	.8	.26
Turnips, raw	20	.3	3.8	2.8	0	25	0	0	–	.04	.05	.6	.1
Watercress	14	tr	.7	3.3	5000	60	0	1.49	–	.1	.1	.6	.1
CHEESE													
Camembert	300	23.2	tr	0	941	0	7.24	8.89	–	.05	.6	.8	.
Cheddar	406	33.5	tr	0	1375	0	12-15	.8	–	.04	.5	.1	.0
Cottage	96	4	1.4	0	137	0	.92	–	–	.02	.19	.08	.0
Edam	304	23	tr	0	941	0	7.16	1.19	–	.04	.4	.06	.0
Mozzarella	252	16	3	0	600	0	12-15	–	–	.018	.3	.1	.0
Stilton	462	40	tr	0	1616	0	12.48	1.49	–	.07	.3	–	
Swiss	369	27	3.4	0	800	0	12-15	–	–	.022	.37	.09	.0
DAIRY													
Goat's Milk	71	4.5	4.6	0	133	1.5	2.4	–	–	.04	.15	.19	.0
Wholemilk	62	3.8	4.7	0	502	1.5	1.52	.18	–	.04	.19	.08	.0
Skim Milk	33	.1	5	0	tr	1.6	tr	tr	–	.04	.2	.08	.0

FOLIC ACID	VIT B12	VIT B5	BIOTIN	CA	P	MG	K	NA	FE	CU	MN	ZN	SE	CR	S	CL
34	0	.2	.7	23	27	8	240	9	.9	.03	-	.2	-	-	-	-
13	0	.1	.4	17	20	12	210	1	.2	.03	-	.2	-	-	-	-
23	0	2	-	3	140	13	470	9	1	.64	-	.1	-	-	34	
-	0	-	-	66	66	27	340	19	1	.12	-	-	-	-	170	
-	0	.02	tr	61	17	22	91	2250	1	.23	-	-	-	-	36	
16	0	.14	.9	31	30	8	140	10	.3	.08	-	.1	-	-	51	
-	0	.3	.4	330	130	52	1080	33	8	.52	-	.9	-	-	-	
67	0	.5	.1	55	69	22	340	17	.6	.1	-	.1	-	-	17	
-	0	.75	.5	15	100	30	340	1	1.9	.23	-	.7	-	-	50	
33	0	2	-	33	270	130	910	38	5.4	.58	-	4	-	-	170	
11	0	.23	-	9	25	11	210	2	.4	.07	-	.2	-	-	-	
8	0	.16	tr	8	39	24	550	6	.6	.15	-	.2	-	-	34	
14	0	.3	.1	8	40	24	570	7	.5	.15	-	.3	-	-	35	
24	0	.18	-	44	27	11	240	59	1.9	.13	-	.1	-	-	38	
140	0	.21	.1	600	93	59	490	120	4	.26	-	.4	-	-	86	
27	0	.11	.1	56	19	11	140	52	.4	.05	-	-	-	-	39	
52	0	.94	-	22	47	13	320	19	.7	.16	-	-	-	-	16	
32	0	.22	-	3	67	23	200	310	.6	.05	-	.6	-	-	-	
52	0	.54	--	4	130	46	300	1	1.1	.16	.02	1.2	.4	.03	-	
.04	0	.17	-	73	24	65	321	86	1.8	-	-	-	-	-	-	
28	0	.33	1.5	13	21	11	290	3	.4	.1	.02	.2	.5	.03	11	
95	0	.38	-	250	60	60	-	-	1.8	-	-	-	-	-	-	
20	0	.2	.1	59	28	7	240	58	.4	.07	-	-	-	-	22	
-	0	.1	.4	220	52	17	310	60	1.6	.14	-	.2	-	-	130	
60	1.2	1.4	6	380	290	17	110	1410	.76	.08	-	3	-	-	-	
20	1.5	.3	1.7	800	520	25	120	610	.4	.03	-	4	-	-	230	
9	.5	-	-	60	140	6	54	450	.1	.02	-	.47	-	-	-	
20	1.4	.3	1.5	740	520	28	160	980	.21	.03	-	4	-	-	670	
9	.8	.08	-	650	460	23	84	470	.2	-	-	3	-	-	-	
-	-	-	-	360	300	27	160	1150	.46	.03	-	-	-	-	230	
6	1.7	.4	-	960	600	36	110	260	.17	-	-	4	11	-	-	
1	tr	.34	2	130	110	20	180	40	.04	.05	-	.3	-	-	-	
5	.3	.35	2	120	95	12	150	50	.05	.02	-	.35	-	-	30	
5	.3	.36	2	130	100	12	150	52	.05	.02	-	.36	-	-	31	

	CAL	FAT	CARBO	FIBRE	VIT A	VIT C	VIT D	VIT E	VIT K	VIT B1	VIT B2	VIT B3 NIACIN	VIT B6
DAIRY—*cont.*													
Buttermilk	41	.9	4.8	0	33	1	–	–	–*	.03	.15	.06	.034
Yoghurt, low fat	52	1	6.2	0	537	.4	tr	.04	–	.05	.26	.12	.04
Butter, salted	740	82	tr	0	3282	tr	30.4	2.98	–	tr	tr	tr	tr
EGGS													
Whole	147	10.9	tr	0	466	0	70	2.38	–	.09	.47	.07	.11
Yolk	339	31	tr	0	1332	0	200	6.85	–	.3	.54	.02	.3
White	36	tr	tr	0	0	0	0	–	–	0	.43	.09	tr
BREAD													
Rye	254	1.1	52	.4	0	0	–	–	–	.18	.07	1.4	.1
Wholemeal	255	2.6	49	1.5	tr	tr	–	.5	–	.3	.1	2.8	.18
CEREALS													
Oatmeal	401	8.7	72.8	7	0	0	0	.15	–	.5	.1	1	.12
Rolled Oats	391	7	68	1.2	0	0	0	.36	20	.6	.14	1	–
Rye	355	1.7	73	2	0	0	0	1.8	–	.4	.22	1.6	–
GRAINS & FLOURS													
Barley	357	1	79	.5	0	0	0	.9	–	.12	.05	3	.22
Buckwheat	347	1	78	–	0	0	–	–	–	0	.04	.4	–
Carob	178	1.11	81	–	–	–	–	–	–	–	–	–	–
Rye Flour	335	2	75.9	–	0	0	0	1.19	–	.4	.22	1	.35
Soya Flour	447	23.5	23.5	11.9	0	0	0	–	–	.75	.31	2	.57
Brown Rice	356	2	77	.9	0	0	0	2	–	.34	.05	5	.55
Wholemeal Flour	318	2	65.8	9.6	0	0	0	1.49	–	.46	.08	5.6	.5
Wheat Bran	353	.4.6	62	9	0	0	0	2.2	–	.7	.35	20	.8
Wheat Germ	395	11	47	2.5	0	0	0	90	–	· 2	.7	4	1.2
Bulgar Wheat	361	1.5	76	1.7	0	0	–	–	–	.3	.15	4	.2
Sago	355	.2	94	–	0	0	0	tr	–	tr	tr	tr	tr
Tapioca	359	.1	95	–	0	0	0	tr	–	tr	tr	tr	tr
FATS & OILS													
Corn Oil	900	100	0	0	0	0	0	28	10	–	–	–	–
Olive Oil	900	100	0	0	0	0	0	20	–	–	–	–	–
Safflower Oil	900	100	0	0	0	0	0	50	–	–	–	–	–
Soy Oil	900	100	0	0	0	0	0	16	–	–	–	–	–

FOLIC ACID	VIT B12	VIT B5	BIOTIN	CA	P	MG	K	NA	FE	CU	MN	ZN	SE	CR	S	CL
-	.22	.28	-	116	89	11	150	100	.05	.005	.01	.4	-	.015	-	
2	tr	-	-	180	140	17	240	76	.09	.04	-	.6	-	-	-	
tr	tr	tr	tr	15	24	2	15	870	.16	.03	-	.15	-	-	9	1340
25	1.7	1.8	25	52	220	12	140	140	2	.1	-	1.5	-	-	180	
52	4.9	4.6	60	130	500	15	120	50	6.1	.3	-	3.6	-	-	170	
1	.1	.3	tr	5	33	11	150	190	.1	.005	-	.03	-	-	180	
23	0	.45	-	75	150	40	145	560	1.6	.017	.5	1.2	-	.06	-	
27	0	.8	2	80	250	80	260	530	2.3	.17	1.2	1.7	70	.06	-	
60	0	1	20	55	380	110	370	33	4.1	.23	-	3	-	-	160	
16	-	-	24	50	400	140	350	2	4.5	-	-	-	-	-	-	
-	-	-	-	40	375	115	470	1	3.7	-	-	-	-	-	-	
20	0	.5	31	16	200	37	160	3	2	-	-	-	66	-	-	
-	-	-	-	11	88	48	320	.91	1	.7	-	-	-	-	-	
-	-	-	-	355	100	-	-	-	-	-	-	-	-	-	-	
78	0	1	6	32	360	92	410	1	2.7	.42	-	2.8	-	-	-	
-	0	1.8	-	210	600	240	1660	1	6.9	-	-	-	-	-	-	
16	0	1.1	12	30	220	90	210	9	1.6	-	-	-	39	-	-	
57	0	.8	7	35	340	140	360	3	4	.4	-	3	-	-	-	
260	0	3	14	120	1300	490	1100	9	15	-	-	-	-	-	-	
330	0	1.2	-	70	1100	340	800	3	9	-	-	-	-	-	-	
-	0	.7	-	30	350	-	230	-	3	-	-	-	-	-	-	
tr	0	tr	tr	10	29	3	5	3	1.2	.03	-	-	-	-	1	
tr	0	tr	tr	8	30	2	20	4	.3	.07	-	-	-	-	4	
-	-	-	-	.18	1.2	.01	-	.04	.4	-	-	-	-	-	-	
-	-	-	-	-	-	-	-	-	-	-	-	-	-	-	-	
-	-	-	-	-	-	-	-	-	-	-	-	-	-	-	-	

	CAL	FAT	CARBO	FIBRE	VIT A	VIT C	VIT D	VIT E	VIT K	VIT B1	VIT B2	VIT B3 NIACIN	VIT B6
NUTS & SEEDS													
Almonds	565	53.5	4.3	14.3	0	tr	0	30	–	.24	.92	2	.1
Brazil Nuts	619	61.5	4.1	9	0	tr	0	9.69	–	1	.12	1.6	.17
Cashew	598	46	29	1.4	100	–	0	–	–	.43	.25	1.8	–
Chestnuts	170	2.7	36.6	6.8	0	tr	0	.75	–	.2	.22	.2	.33
Hazelnuts	380	36	6.8	6.1	0	tr	0	31.29	–	.4	–	.9	.55
Walnuts	525	51.5	5	5.2	0	tr	0	1.19	–	.3	.13	1	.73
Pumpkin Seeds	552	46.5	15	–	70	–	–	–	–	.24	.19	2.39	–
Sesame Seeds	582	53.5	18	–	–	–	–	–	–	.18	.13	5.39	–
Sunflower Seeds	599	47	20	4	50	–	0	–	–	2	.23	5.4	1.3
MISCELLANEOUS													
Yeast, Brewers													
Debittered	317	1	38	1.7	tr	tr	–	–	–	16	4	40	2500
Cod Liver Oil	899	99.8	0	0	59940	0	–	–	–	0	0	0	0
Cider Vinegar	20	0	90	0	–	–	–	–	–	–	–	–	–
Molasses, blackstrap	860	–	220	0	–	–	–	–	–	.02	.8	8	1
Maple Syrup	1000	0	260	0	0	0	–	–	–	–	–	0	–
Kelp	–	1.09	.4	0	–	–	–	–	–	–	.33	5.7	–
Soybean Milk	33.04	1.48	2.22	0	40	0	–	–	–	.08	.03	.2	–
Honey, comb	281	4.6	74.4	–	0	tr	0	–	–	tr	.05	.2	–
in jars	288	tr	76.4	–	0	tr	0	–	–	tr	.05	.2	–

FOLIC ACID	VIT B12	VIT B5	BIOTIN	CA	P	MG	K	NA	FE	CU	MN	ZN	SE	CR	S	CL
96	0	.47	.4	250	440	260	860	6	4.2	.14	-	3.1	-	-	150	
-	0	.23	-	180	590	410	760	2	2.8	1.1	-	4.2	-	-	290	
70	0	1.3	-	40	375	270	460	15	4	-	-	-	-	-	-	
-	0	.47	1.3	46	74	33	500	11	.9	.23	-	-	-	-	29	
72	0	1.15	-	44	230	56	350	1	1.1	.21	-	2.4	-	-	75	
66	0	.9	2	61	510	130	690	3	2.4	.31	-	3	-	-	100	
-	-	-	-	51	1143	-	-	-	11.3	-	-	-	-	-	-	
-	-	-	-	110	592	181	-	-	2.39	1.61	-	-	-	-	-	
-	0	1.4	-	120	800	40	920	30	7	5	.4	11	71	.007	-	
3900	0	12000	110	200	1750	230.	1900	120	17	5.3	.4	11	71	.007	-	
0	0	tr	tr	tr	tr	tr	tr	tr	tr	tr	tr	tr	tr	tr	tr	tr
-	-	-	-	6	9.3	-	100	.67	.6	-	-	-	-	-	-	
.04	0	1.8	36	2740	340	1032	11700	380	64.5	-	-	-	-	-	-	
-	-	-	-	420	32	-	700	40	4.8	-	-	-	-	-	-	
-	-	-	-	1093	240	.08	5273	3007	.1	tr	-	-	-	-	-	
-	-	-	-	21	48	-	-	.78	-	-	-	-	-	-	-	
-	0	-	-	8	32	2	35	7	.2	.04	-	-	-	-	1	
-	0	-	-	5	17	2	51	11	.4	.05	-	-	-	-	1	

Key

Ca – Calcium   P – Phosphorus   Mg – Magnesium   K – Potassium
Na – Sodium   Fe – Iron   Cu – Copper   Mn – Manganese   Zn – Zinc
Se – Selenium   Cr – Chromium   S – Sulphur   Cl – Chlorine

Useful Addresses

GREEN FARM NUTRITION CENTRE For details of our information services, nutritional advisory service, *Green Farm Magazine*, books, health catalogue, offprint services, clinics, courses (home study, residential and one day), travelling audio-visual shows and open days please send a second class stamp to the Green Nutrition Centre, Burwash Common, East Sussex TN19 7LX. Tel: 0435 882180.

ACTION AGAINST ALLERGY Amelia Hill, 43 The Downs, London SW20. Tel: 01-947 5082.
Information and advice if you think you have allergies.

BRITISH GOAT SOCIETY Miss A. Bell, Blacknest Lodge, Sunninghill, Ascot, Berks. Tel: Ascot 24666. Advice on goat's milk products and producers.

BRITISH SOCIETY FOR NUTRITIONAL MEDICINE Information Officer, Dr Alan Stewart, 5 Somerhill Road, Hove, East Sussex, BN3 1RP.

CHEMICAL-FREE ANIMAL FEED SUPPLIERS Allen & Page Ltd, Quality Mills, Norwich, NR3 1SA. Tel: 0603 620237. Suppliers of chemical-free animal feeds. Contact: Ben Page.

DAYS FARM NATURAL FOODS Lippitts Hill, High Beach, Loughton, Essex. Tel: 01-502 2621. Will deliver quality organic fruit and vegetables, meat, additive-free eggs, bread, cakes, grains, nuts, cheese etc. throughout the London area, and will tell you who can help you if they can't.

FOODWATCH (Mail order foods and advice) Peter Campbell, Butts Pond Industrial Estate, Sturminster Newton, Dorset DT10 1OZ. Tel: 0258 73356.

HENRY DOUBLEDAY RESEARCH ASSOCIATION Ryton on Dunsmore, Coventry CV8 3LG. Advice on all aspects of organic gardening (particular interest in comfrey and its uses). Offers a regular newsletter, membership and catalogue of seeds, books, fertilisers, etc.

INFINITY FOODS 25 North Street, Brighton BN1 1YA. Tel: 0273 424 060. Free deliveries for orders over £100 in Kent, Sussex, Hants, Oxfordshire and London (so get an order together with friends). Will also send by carrier anywhere in the country or even abroad. First class organic grains, nuts, beans, teas, bread etc. Very large selection.

NATIONAL SOCIETY FOR RESEARCH INTO ALLERGY P.O. Box 45 Hinckley, Leics. LE10 1JY. Membership and regular newsletter.

NATURAL HEALTH NETWORK 1 Caxton House, Caxton, Limpsfield Chart, Surrey RH8 0TD. Tel: 01-499 1542. Will put you in touch with courses, events and services in your area.

ORGANIC BUTCHER 217 Holloway Road, London N7. Tel: 01-609 7016. Additive-free and organic meats delivered throughout London and sent all over the country by train.

ORGANIC CHEESES M. Deauville, New Health Farm, Acton, Newcastle, Staffs. Tel. 0278 680 366. They will mail to you if your order is large enough or tell you where your nearest stockist is.

ORGANIC FARM FOOD Unit 7, Ellerslie, Lyham Road, London SW2. Tel: 01-274 0234. Wholesale suppliers (so persuade your greengrocer to buy from them). You can also buy in person if you live near enough.

ORGANIC FOOD GUIDE lists all known sources of organic foods throughout the country accurate at time of going to press, available from the Henry Doubleday Research Association at the above address price £2.50 plus 50p post and packing.

ORGANIC WINES AND CIDER West Heath Wine, West Heath, Pirbright, Surrey GU24 0QE. Tel: 04867 6464. Free deliveries to London postal districts. Ask if they can send to you by rail or carrier.

PESTICIDES ACTION NETWORK c/o Friends of the Earth, 377 City Road, London EC1.

SOIL ASSOCIATION Walnut Tree Manor, Haughley, Stowmarket, Suffolk. Tel: 0449 70235. Advice on all aspects of organic gardening and farming.

WHOLEFOOD SHOP 24 Paddington Street, London W1. Tel: 01-935 3924. Organic grains, nuts, dried fruit, beans, juices, etc. and some fresh foods can be sent all over the country.

References

PART I

2 The Lost Instinct

1 Stitt Paul A. *Fighting the Food Giants*. Natural Press, Manitowoc, WI. 54220

2 MacGregor G. *The Salt Free Diet Book*. Positive Health Guide, Dunitz 1985

3 Information Officer, British Society for Nutritional Medicine, 5 Somerhill Road, Hove, East Sussex BN3 1RP

4 Murphy, J. V. Intoxication following ingestion of elemental zinc. *J. Amer. Med. Assoc.* 212: 2119–2120, 1970

5 *Manual of Nutrition*. HMSO 1976

6 Colgan M. *Your Personal Vitamin Profile*. Blond and Briggs 1983

7 *Recommended Dietary Allowances*. National Academy of Sciences, Washington 1980

8 Price W. *Nutrition and Physical Degeneration*. Price Pottenger Foundation, P.O. Box 2614, La Mesa, California 92041, 1979

9 Davis, C. M. Self selection of diet by newly weaned infants. *Amer. J. of Diseases of Children* Vol 36, 4 Oct 1928

3 The Wright Direction

1 Milne A. *The World of Christopher Robin*. Methuen 1977

2 Stare F. and McWilliams M. *Living Nutrition*. 2nd Edition John Wiley 1977

3 Trowell H. *'Hunter Gatherers'* in *Western Diseases*. Ed. Burkitt D. and Trowell H., Edward Arnold, 1981, page 14

4 Lee R. 'What hunters do for a living' in *Man the Hunter*, 30 – 48. Ed. R. B. Lee and I . Devore. Aldine, Chicago, 1968

5 Washburn S. and Lancaster C. in *Man the Hunter*, 303. Eds R. B Lee and I. Devore. Aldine, Chicago, 1968

6 Schauss A. *Diet, Crime and Delinquency*. Parker House, 2340 Parker St, Berkeley, California

7 Ogle J. *The Stop Smoking Diet*. Piatkus, London, 1981

8 Muggeo M., Bar R. S. and Roth J. Change in affinity of insulin

receptors following oral glucose in normal adults. *J. Clin. Endocrinol. Metab.* 44: 1206, 1977

9 Faludi G., Bendersky G. and Gerber P. *Annals of the New York Academy of Sciences*, Vol 148, 26 March 1968

10 Harper C. United Airlines, quoted in *New Dynamics of Preventive Medicine*, Stratton, New York, Vol 3, 1975

11 Unpublished data from *1966/67 National Health Interview Survey*, USA

12 Atkins R. *Dr Atkins' Superenergy Diet*. Corgi 1978

13 Carson Rachel *Silent Spring*. Crest, Greenwich, Connecticut, 1962

14 Association of Public Analysts Report 1984 quoted in *The Sunday Times*

15 Pesticides Action Network c/o Friends of the Earth, 377 City Road, London EC1

16 *Pesticides: The case of an industry out of control*. Report available from Friends of the Earth, 377 City Road, London EC1

17 Pfeiffer C. *Mental and Elemental Nutrients*. Keats, Connecticut, USA, 1975

18 Smoked Meat and Diabetes. *World Medicine*, Vol 19, 8. 21 Jan 1984

19 Schell O. *Modern Meat*. Random House 1978

20 Shahani K., Reddy A., Joe A. Nutritional and therapeutic aspects of cultured dairy products. *Proc 19th Intern'l Dairy Cong.*, Vol 1e, 569 – 570

21 Pearce F. and Cherfas J. Antibiotics breed lethal poisons. *New Scientist*, 13 Sept 1984

22 Downing D. Address given to British Naturopathic and Osteopathic Assoc., 6 Oct 1984

23 Crook W. *The Yeast Connection*. Professional Books 1984

24 Schoental R. Health hazards of secondary metabolites of fusarium *Microbiologie – Aliments – Nutrition* 1983, Vol 1, 101 – 107

25 Henderson B. et al. Endogenous hormones as a major factor in human cancer. *Cancer Res.*, 42, 3232 – 3239, 1982

26 Ministry of Agriculture, Fisheries, and Food. *Manual of Nutrition*. HMSO 1976

27 Kenton L. *Raw Energy*. Century, London, 1984

28 Ganong W. *Review of Medical Physiology*. Lange, California, 1969

29 Kunz-Bircher R. *Bircher Benner Health Guide*. Woodbridge Press, Santa Barbara, California

30 Dodwell C. Personal letter. 5/11/1984

31 Sugimura T. and Sato S. *Cancer Res*. (Suppl.) 43, 2415s, 1983

32 Sugimura T. and Nagao M. in *Mutagenicity: New Horizons in Genetic Toxicology*, J. A. Heddle, Ed. Academic Press, New York, 1982, pp 77 – 78

33 Shorland F. B. et al., *J. Agric. Food Chem.* 29, 863, 1981

34 Pryor W. A. Ed., *Free Radicals in Biology*. Academic Press, New York, 1976 to 1982, Vols 1 to 5

35 Stich H. F., Rosin M. P. et al. in *Mutagenicity: New Horizons in Genetic Toxicology*, J. A. Heddle, Ed. Academic Press, New York, 1982, pp, 117 – 142

36 Trichopoulos D. et al. *Int. J. Cancer* 28, 691, 1981

37 Ames B. N. Dietary carcinogens and anticarcinogens. *Science*, Vol 221, 23 Sept 1983

38 Pearson D. and Shaw S. *Life Extension*. Warner Books, USA, 1982

39 Hopkins Tanne J. *American Health*. 2(5), p 48, 1983

40 Henry Doubleday Association. *Newsletter*. Summer 1984

41 Schauss A. *Body Chemistry and behaviour*. St Bartholomew's Hospital, 17–18 Nov 1984

42 Boyd Eaton S. and Konner M. Paleolithic Nutrition. *New England J. Med.*, Vol 312, 5, 31 Jan 1985

43 Mandell M. *Dr Mandell's 5 Day Allergy Relief System*. Arrow 1983

44 *Food Additives – Are the risks worthwhile?* Ecoropa, Crickhowell, Powys, Wales, NP8 1TA. Sent free if you send an S.A.E.

45 Hanssen M. *E for Additives*. Thorsons, Northants, 1984

46 Jacobson M. *Eater's Digest. The Consumer's Factbook of Food Additives*. Anchor Press, Doubleday, 1976, and private communication Eric Millstone Ph.D., Sussex University

47 Schauss A. *Diet, Crime and Delinquency*. Parker House, 2340 Parker St, Berkeley, California

48 Grant D. and Joice J. *Food Combining for Health*. Thorsons 1984

49 Pavlov A. *The Work of the Digestive Glands*. Charles Griffin 1910

50 Discussed at British Society for Nutritional Medicine conference, Sept 1984

51 MacGregor G. *The Salt Free Diet Book*. Positive Health Guide, Dunitz 1984

52 Price W. *Nutrition and Physical Degeneration*. Price Pottenger Foundation, P. O. Box 2614, La Mesa, California 92041, 1979

53 Philpott W. and Kalita D. *Brain Allergies*. Keats Publishing, New Canaan, Connecticut, 1980

54 Wright J. *Dr Wright's Healing with Nutrition*. Rodale Press 1984

PART 2

1 Atkins R. Exhaustion, Causes and Treatment. Quoted in *Dr Atkins' Superenergy Diet*. Corgi 1978

2 Burkitt D. & Trowell H. *Western Diseases*. Edward Arnold 1981

3 Glass, A., Burman, K. & Boehm, 'Endocrine function and obesity', *Metabolism,* 30, 89, 1982

4 Glick Z. & Brag G. 'Brown Adipose Tissue: Thermic Response Increased by a Single Low Protein, High Carbohydrate Meal', *Science*, 213, 1125, 1982; Moulopoulos S. 'Metabolic Insufficiency as a Limiting Factor in Obesity', *Hormones and Metabolic research*, 13, 477, 1982

5 Bland J. *Your Personal Health Programme*. Thorsons 1985

6 Baba N. & Hashim S. 'Enhanced thermogenesis and diminished deposition of fat in response to a diet containing medium chain triglyceride', *Amer. J. Clin. Nutr.* 35, 678, 1982

7 Sharif N. and MacDonald I. 'Differences in Dietary-Induced Thermogenesis with Various Carbohydrates in Overweight Men', *Amer. J. Clin. Nutr.* 35, 267, 1982

8 Levine S. *Food Addiction, Food Allergy and Overweight*. Allergy Research Group, 2336-C Stanwell Circle, Concord, Calif 94520. Published in *Bestways* magazine

9 Abraham G. Nutritional Factors in the Etiology of the Premenstrual Tension Syndrome. *J. Reproductive Med.*, Vol 28, number 7, July 1983

10 Abraham G. Magnesium Deficiency in premenstrual tension. *Magnesium Bulletin* 4:68, 1982

11 Muggeo M., Bar R.S., Roth J: Change in affinity of insulin receptors following oral glucose in normal adults. *J. Clin. Endocrinol. Metab.* 44: 1206, 1977

12 DePirro R, Fusco A, Bertoli A, et al. Insulin receptors during the menstrual cycle in normal women. *J. Clin. Endocrinol. Metab.* 47:1387, 1978

13 Report by Dr J. P. Minton in *JAMA Medical News* 24, 1221, 1979

14 Check W. Benign breast lumps may regress with change in diet. *J. Amer. Med. Assoc.* 23 March 1979, p 1221

15 London R. S et al. Endocrine parameters and a-tocopherol therapy of patients with mammary dysplasia. *Cancer Res.*, pp 3811–3813, Sept. 1981

16 Gonzalez E. Vitamin E relieves most cystic breast disease. *Medical News*, 5 Sept 1980

17 Marathon effort takes king of the road into history. *Daily Mail*, 3 May 1983

PART 3

1 Burkitt D. & Trowell H. *Western Diseases*. Edward Arnold 1981

Recommended Reading

Here is a list of interesting and informative reading. All of these are available from the Green Farm Bookshop by mail order if you can't obtain them locally.

America the Poisoned. Lewis Regenstein. Acropolis Books Ltd, Washington DC.

The Colon Cleansing Handbook. Brian Wright. Green Press.

Diet, Crime and Delinquency. Alexander Schauss. Parker House 2340, Parker Street, Berkeley, California 94704.

Dig for Survival. How to grow your own organic foods. Send 25p in stamps to the Henry Doubleday Research Association, Ryton on Dunsmore, Coventry, CV8 3LG.

Food Additives, Are the Risks Worthwhile? Very informative free leaflet from Ecoropa, Crickhowell, Powys, Wales, NP8 1TA. Send them an S.A.E.

Food Combining for Health. Doris Grant and J. Joice. Thorsons 1984.

The Green Farm Magazine. Details from the Green Farm Nutrition Centre, Burwash Common, East Sussex TN19 7LX. Tel: 0435 882180.

Heal Yourself Naturally. Brian Wright. Century Hutchinson 1986

The Herbal Combinations Handbook. Brian Wright. Green Press 1984.

The Hyperactive Child. Belinda Barnes and Irene Colquhoun. Thorsons 1984.

Illustrated Physiology. McNaught and Callander. Churchill Livingstone 1975.

Look Again at the Label. A special report by the Soil Association with a very helpful explanation of and guide to the E numbers (now given to EEC food additives and commonly found on packaged food). Available for 65p including postage from The Soil Association, Walnut Tree Manor, Haughley, Stowmarket, Suffolk 1P14 3RS.

A Month by Month Guide to Organic Gardening. Laurence D. Hills. Thorsons.

Nutrition and Vitamin Therapy. Michael Lesser M. D. Thorsons.

Nutrition Handbook. Brian and Celia Wright. Green Press, New Edition 1985.

Nutrition Programmes Handbook. Brian and Celia Wright. Green Press.

Raw Energy. Leslie Kenton. Century 1984

Sprout for the Love of Everybody. Victoras Kulvinskas. Omango d'Press.

Your Health Under Siege. Jeffrey Bland Ph.D. The Stephen Green Press, Brattleboro, Vermont, USA.

Your Personal Health Programme. Jeffrey Bland Ph.D. Thorsons.

Index